W
84
1wk

NHS Reforms

imposing control?

NICE, CHI and the NHS Reforms
Enabling excellence or imposing control?

Edited by

Professor Andrew Miles MSc MPhil PhD
Professor of Health Services Research and Director,
University of East London Centre for Health Services Research
at St Bartholomew's Hospital, London

Professor John R Hampton MA DM DPhil FRCP FESC FFPM
Professor of Cardiology,
Cardiovascular Medicine,
University Hospital, Nottingham

Professor Brian Hurwitz MA MSc MD MRCGP FRCP
Professor of Primary Care and General Practice,
Imperial College of Science, Technology and Medicine, London

UeL University Centre for
Health Services Research

AESCULAPIUS MEDICAL PRESS
LONDON SAN FRANCISCO SYDNEY

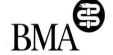

Published by

Aesculapius Medical Press (London, San Francisco, Sydney)
UeL University Centre for Health Services Research
St Bartholomew's Hospital
London
EC1A 7BE

British Library Cataloguing in Publication Data

A catalogue record for this book is available from the British Library

ISBN 1 903044 06 5

Further copies of this volume are available from:

Claudio Melchiorri
Research Dissemination Fellow
UeL Centre for Health Services Research
St Bartholomew's Hospital
London EC1A 7BE

Fax: 0171 601 7085
e-mail: cmelchiorri@mds.qmw.ac.uk

Typeset, printed and bound in Britain by
Peter Powell Origination & Print Limited

Contents

Contributors

Alan Alderson, Chief Physicist, Kent Cancer Centre

Anita Burrell, Manager of Health Economics, Aventis Pharma UK, West Malling, Kent

Bruce G Charlton MD, Visiting Professor in Health Services Research, UeL Centre for Health Services Research, St Bartholomew's Hospital, London, and Department of Psychology, University of Newcastle, Newcastle upon Tyne

Ian Dodds-Smith MA(Cantab), Partner and Head of Healthcare Law Group, CMS Cameron McKenna, Solicitors, City of London, London

George Dowswell BSc(Econ) PhD, Principal Research Fellow, Nuffield Institute for Health, University of Leeds, Leeds

Gene Feder BSc(Hons) MB BS MD FRCGP, Professor of Primary Care Research and Development, Department of General Practice, St Bartholomew's and the Royal London School of Medicine and Dentistry, Queen Mary & Westfield College, London

Neville W Goodman DPhil FRCA, Consultant Anaesthetist, Southmead Hospital, Bristol

David G Grahame-Smith CBE MB BS PhD FRCP, Rhodes Professor of Clinical Pharmacology, and Honorary Consultant Physician in General Internal Medicine and Clinical Pharmacology, Radcliffe Infirmary, Oxford

John R Hampton MA DM DPhil FRCP FESC FFPM, Professor of Cardiology, Queens Medical Centre, University Hospital, Nottingham

Stephen Harrison BSc(Econ) MPhil PhD, Professor of Health Policy and Politics, Nuffield Institute for Health, University of Leeds, Leeds

Brian Hurwitz MA MSc MD MRCGP FRCP, Professor of Primary Care and General Practice, Imperial College of Science, Technology and Medicine, London

Daniel Jackson, Health Economist, Aventis Pharma UK, West Malling, Kent

Roger D James MD FRCP, Clinical Director, Kent Cancer Network, & Professor of Clinical Oncology

Michael Loughlin PhD, Lecturer in Philosophy, Department of Humanities & Applied Social Studies, Manchester Metropolitan University, Alsager, Manchester

Michael Power PhD ACA ATII, PD Leake Professor of Accounting, & Director of the Centre for the Analysis of Risk and Regulation, London School of Economics and Political Science, London

Michael Vaile MD, Director of Public Health, West Kent Health Authority, Kent

Philip D Welsby FRCP(Ed), Consultant Physician, Infectious Diseases Unit, Western General Hospital, Edinburgh

Preface

The present volume documents the debate and recommendations of a major national symposium planned jointly between The British Medical Association and the University of East London Centre for Health Services Research, held at The Royal College of Physicians in London on 9 September 1999. The volume, updated in March 2000, aims systematically to address twelve principal areas of focus relating to the National Institute for Clinical Excellence (NICE) and the Commission for Health Improvement (CHI), two recent innovations in the National Health Service of the United Kingdom that have precipitated a wide range of scientific and clinical concerns.

It is not our intention here to provide a thorough commentary on each of the constituent chapters, which we believe to speak lucidly and elegantly for themselves. We acknowledge, however, that many of the points made in the current volume may prove immediately contentious among those who accept the need for NICE and CHI as unquestionable, and who may view doubts about the utility and necessity of these institutions as problems only for the doubters. The philosophies of NICE, which draw on principles of evidence-based medicine and considerations of cost, and those of CHI, based on principles of external inspection and enforcement, certainly stand in acute contrast to the established nature of health service organisation and delivery and to the practice of the majority of clinicians.

Rather than focusing selectively on those aspects of NICE and CHI likely to prove beneficial in the NHS and which have been treated extensively elsewhere, the present volume, in a series of constructive analyses, seeks to present frank and penetrating discussion of some of the likely limitations and dangers of these institutions. We welcome such activity, it is in the nature of science. In this spirit we publish the present volume and commend its use in the advancement of an open, balanced and intellectually rigorous debate.

Andrew Miles MSc MPhil PhD
John R Hampton MA DM DPhil FRCP FESC FFPM
Brian Hurwitz MA MSc MD MRCGP FRCP

London 10 March 2000

The views expressed herein are those of the authors alone and do not necessarily represent the official views of The British Medical Association and the Universities of East London, Nottingham or London.

Chapter 1

'Quality' and 'excellence': meaning versus rhetoric

Michael Loughlin

> *'The British government has committed itself to a programme of enhancing the quality of care given to National Health Service (NHS) patients.'*
> (Rawlins 1999, p.1079)

> *'No-one is opposed to quality. How could anyone be ...?'*
> (Curtis 1993, p.191)

Introduction

It would indeed seem absurd to be opposed to quality and excellence. It surely follows that we should all welcome the British Government's 'commitment' to these things, as evidenced by the creation of a national institute to promote clinical excellence in the NHS.

I must immediately betray my own academic background, almost certainly inviting derision in the process, by responding that it depends on what one *means* by 'quality' and 'excellence'. Those of us who are philosophers by trade or inclination are well aware that critical reflection upon the meanings of terms has very much fallen out of fashion in contemporary discussions of all matters of practical importance. The merest acquaintance with the vast literature produced by the powers-that-be (in Government and in NHS management) concerning health services delivery and organisation is sufficient to confirm the view of one prominent management specialist that such 'intellectual ruminations' are deemed 'not to our purpose' (Wall 1994, p.318). Texts and journal articles (indeed, whole journals) are dedicated to the discussion of concepts which, it soon becomes clear, the authors of the texts and the contributors to the journals have expended no intellectual energy whatsoever in attempting to analyse. (Useful illustrations are Joss & Kogan (1995), any of the contributions to Al-Assaf & Schemele (1993) or any contribution to the *International Journal of Health Care Quality Assurance*.)

It is perhaps worth pausing for a moment to consider what this tells us about the 'intellectual environment' within the developed nations at the turn of the millennium. A person who uses a tool or mechanism for some important purpose, but who never troubles to think about how it works, or whether he or she is using it correctly, is usually thought of as an idiot. When that tool is the language in terms of which we conceptualise and evaluate practices we regard as vital to our common well-being, the person who disdains critical thought is called a 'pragmatist'.

The joint development of the new National Institute for Clinical Excellence (NICE) and its associate body – the Commission for Health Improvement (CHI) – is heralded by their proponents as a significant change in the way we will understand and conduct health service activity in future.[1] One of the roles of NICE will be to appraise new technologies, effectively vetting those deemed ineffective, or too costly, or otherwise inappropriate for use in the NHS. It would surely be remarkable, then, if the advocates of the new institution opposed subjecting *its* methods and assumptions to critical scrutiny before employing them to transform the service. What is the basis for the claim that this new way of promoting 'excellence' is likely to be effective? How will the Institute conceptualise 'clinical excellence' and its relationship with such things as knowledge, evidence, variation in practice, judgement, interpretation, rationality, science and value? Do the proponents of NICE *have* a well-worked-out and defensible account of these concepts and the relationships between them? Is it one that they would care to explain in detail and debate with those practitioners most likely to be affected by the Institute's existence? What conception of good practice is embodied *by the very idea* that one promotes it via a central organisation? If that idea should turn out *not* to be defensible, what are the implications for the conceptual foundations of both NICE and CHI? There is nothing 'pragmatic' about changing direction without pausing to study a map. It is still less pragmatic (in any worthwhile sense of the word) to plan one's journey with reference to a map whose accuracy one has taken no measures to confirm.

The need for conceptual analysis

Underlying any attempt to *improve* practice in a given area is some conception of what it means to do well in that context, and this conception is likely to be grounded in a set of assumptions about the nature of the context, the goals of the practices in question, and more general beliefs about the nature of value which make sense of the claim that the practice's goals are worthwhile in the first place. All practical thinking, even about relatively straightforward matters, takes place against the background of a fairly sophisticated conceptual 'map': a picture of the world and our place within it which we develop over the course of our lives and which, if we are at all reflective, is continually being adapted in response to new information. Even the simple judgement that I would be best off taking a particular route home presupposes a set of related beliefs about the possible options open to me, the obstacles I am likely to encounter at specific points, the relative value of getting home faster as weighed against the value of taking a more 'scenic' route, and so forth. These beliefs themselves are given sense with reference to general beliefs about the nature of the world and what matters

---

1   Many would argue that it does not so much represent a change as the logical conclusion of a movement towards greater managerial control of clinical practice which has been gaining momentum for several years. The development of an organisation such as NICE was predicted by one astute author in 1993 (Charlton 1993).

in life. I may rarely stop to reflect upon the more fundamental of these background assumptions, but they are there, nonetheless. This is surely all the more obvious in the case of the judgements I form about important matters of public policy, where more complicated issues are at stake and where there is no broad consensus about what is right, nor even about how to begin determining this. Indeed, the reason why debates about such matters often seem so intractable is precisely because the parties involved bring with them different underlying assumptions, ones which they fail to subject to critical attention and which they frequently fail to articulate, or even to recognise (Loughlin AJ 1998, pp.62–6).

To do philosophy is to examine such underlying assumptions: it is to bring them into the foreground, to *make* them the subject of critical attention. The process of discovering underlying assumptions is called conceptual analysis. The very fact that certain claims seem plausible, or that certain inferences seem valid, can indicate the existence of a set of assumptions which may or may not stand up to scrutiny. There may be commitments implicit within the questions I think it appropriate to ask, what I think *requires* explanation and what (by implication) I treat as part of an uncontentious background, requiring no special account. If we are to develop adequate defences of our views about any controversial issue, it is necessary, at least, to be aware of what they commit us to, since we may find that we are otherwise committed to ideas that we could not defend when spelled out in detail.

Elsewhere I have characterised an 'ideologue' as a person who views his or her own assumptions as sheer common sense, too obvious to be worth debating (Loughlin M 1996a). For such a person the only questions worthy of serious attention are 'pragmatic', concerning how one moves from (one's own) theory to practice. The philosopher and the ideologue are natural enemies. The latter views the former's obsession with spelling out assumptions clearly, and subjecting them to critical analysis, as an irritating distraction from the 'practical' business of turning (one's own) ideas into reality. Such intellectual reflection can be dismissed as an 'academic exercise', of no interest to those immersed in the 'real world' – a place where, apparently, everyone is far too busy implementing the latest idea to have time to assess the question of its worth.

The real effect of setting up a dichotomy between the 'intellectual' and the 'practical' is not, of course, to make one's thinking more 'practical'. Rather, it is to protect one set of ideas – normally the one behind the most fashionable or dominant approaches to practice – from criticism, by ruling the practice of rigorous intellectual criticism 'out of court'. Such a mentality smacks not so much of pragmatism but of bigotry and intellectual repression. The refusal to explain clearly what one means is *at best* a recipe for confusion. Far from being an alternative to practical thinking, if thinking is to provide the basis for coherent practice, it is essential that logical confusions about the meanings of terms and the implications of statements are avoided through conceptual analysis. The choice is not between academic and practical thinking, but between clear practical thinking and confused practical thinking, and only the dishonest can profit from the prevalence of confusion.

Bearing this in mind, we have reason to be disturbed by the recent history of the NHS. For more than a decade successive administrations have introduced a series of management reforms to the service. Unsurprisingly (but nonetheless remarkably), these changes were motivated by a range of political and ideological considerations, rather than systematic reflection upon the nature and purpose of the organisation itself. Although terms such as 'quality', 'excellence', and 'value' abound, and some commentators are even prepared to talk at length about the 'value-base' of the NHS (IHSM 1993), its 'theoretical framework' and 'ultimate purpose' (*ibid*. p14; Liddle 1992, p.1), as well as the 'goals' and 'criteria' which allegedly 'underpin' all health service activity (Peters 1992; Berwick 1993; IHSM 1993, p.23; Laffel & Blumenthal 1993; Joss & Kogan 1995, p.53), there is little in the way of detailed explanation, let alone defence, of the specific uses being made of these terms in support of the particular policies and practices advocated. It seems that authors are willing to plunder the *language* of philosophy and the sciences, making frequent reference to 'general principles', 'axioms', 'theoretical models', 'paradigm-shifts' and a large number of concepts with an evaluative component to their meaning (including, in addition to those already mentioned, 'equity', 'need' and 'well-being') but typically they fail to take on board the *methods* of these subjects, eschewing intellectual rigour and even the basic requirements of clarity and logical consistency (Loughlin M 1994a, 1994b, 1996a; Miles *et al.* 1995).

Instead, it is generally thought sufficient to 'defend' a policy by the repeated use of positive evaluative terminology – hence the mantra-like repetition of the buzzwords 'quality' and 'excellence' in so many government and management documents – without supplying any account of the criteria which justify their use in a given context. Then, having 'established' (purely by verbal association) that one's favoured policy represents or gives rise to 'excellence', it is usual to discuss at length the problems in *implementing* that approach. Since anyone opposed to one's view is now taken (by definition) to be opposed to quality or excellence, authors think it reasonable to conceptualise such dissent as a 'problem' to be overcome (rather than a legitimate expression of independent thought, deserving a clear and well-thought-out *answer*) and to diagnose the problem with reference to the massive ignorance or even the 'psychological needs' of the dissenter (see Heginbotham 1993; Merry 1993, pp.57–8; Joss & Kogan 1995, p.43. I discuss the Orwellian flavour of this style of 'argument' in a little more detail in Loughlin M 1993, 1996a.)

This situation is not a matter of 'mere' academic concern. One of the reasons we employ evaluative language is to affect the attitudes, and consequently the behaviour, of others (Loughlin M 1993; Stevenson 1944). If I successfully affect people's attitudes purely by the use of persuasive language, without providing them with any *good reasons* to accept what I am saying, then in a very real sense I undermine their status as rational, autonomous beings. The alternative to thinking critically about one's fundamental assumptions is to allow one's ideas and attitudes, and ultimately one's behaviour, to be shaped by forces which one fails even to perceive, let alone control. If that is my condition, it makes very little sense to speak of me as a person who 'thinks for himself'. A political culture which derides critical reflection is an ideologue's paradise. It is no coincidence that the decline in the fortunes of philosophy (and other academic disciplines aimed at improving the quality and rigour of human thought) has been accompanied by the rise in influence and status of the political spin-doctor, whose science is the manipulation of an intellectually disempowered populace. The fact that, in certain policy circles, the terms 'intellectual' and 'academic' are typically used pejoratively testifies to the shameless intellectual poverty of contemporary culture. That the expression 'on-message' can be employed openly, without causing a scandal, shows how far along the road to institutionalised stupidity and intellectual repression we have already moved.

In such an environment, philosophical analysis is a necessary form of intellectual and moral self-defence. Judging by the style and tone of large portions of the literature produced by government and management organisations, it appears that the ideologues of New Britain are intent upon taking every evaluative term and making it their own, leaving no language in terms of which their favoured doctrines can be *persuasively* criticised.[2] We have become so accustomed to nonsense that we barely notice the violence being done to our language on a regular basis, yet like any mechanism, the more you misuse it, the less likely it is to work well in future. (As a philosopher, I struggle to achieve an *adequate* understanding of most of the problems I confront, but it seems that managers and politicians achieve 'excellence' every time they put pen to paper.) More than ever, it is imperative that we ask of those in positions of power in public life: 'What do you mean?' What is it that *justifies* the uses they make of terminology and the conclusions they draw? We must insist upon being given a serious and well-thought-out answer. To waive the right to have these questions taken seriously is potentially to give away so much more.

The meaning of 'quality' and 'excellence'

What, then, do the defenders of NICE and CHI mean by the terms 'quality' and 'excellence'? What conception of good practice underlies their expressed confidence that the creation of these bodies, and the 'clinical governance strategy' of which they are a part, will 'improve the quality of care that is given to patients in the NHS' (Rawlins 1999, p.1082)? Crucially, have they explained their assumptions and

---

2 To oppose the dominant ethos is, by definition, to oppose quality, equity, meeting needs, patient autonomy, well-being … in short, all things good. Consider how quickly and easily the language of 'empowerment', initially popular with certain radical critics of the political *status quo*, was assimilated by the management vocabulary of the NHS and used to justify the imposition of unfamiliar working practices upon a sceptical workforce. Since dissent is regarded as a problem for the dissenter, one 'empowers' the dissenter by persuading her to accept that one's favoured approach is the 'way forward', thus 'enabling' her to participate in the 'quality revolution' (Loughlin M 1996a).

supplied any convincing *arguments* in support of them? Without clear arguments at the conceptual level, it is meaningless to say that we have been given any *good reasons* to accept their statements – and the attempt to impose any form of 'governance' upon a working population *without* providing that population with good reasons to accept it will be experienced by its members as a form of oppression, and rightly resisted.

The best evidence available to help us reconstruct the thinking behind NICE comes from the statements made by its defenders. In an article in *The Lancet*, the chairman of NICE, Professor Sir Michael Rawlins (1999), outlined the aims and functions of the new institute and detailed the concerns which led to its creation. In addition to the already-mentioned role of appraising new and existing health technologies, Rawlins lists as the key functions of NICE the promotion of clinical audit and the development of clinical guidelines. The main concerns seem to be that all decisions in the health service should be made on the basis of sound evidence, that 'unexplained' variations in the way patients are treated should be eliminated where possible, and that treatments employed should be cost-effective. To help achieve this, NICE will provide 'a single, authoritative source of advice' to health professionals and their managers. While this advice 'will not be mandatory' (it is not really clear that it could meaningfully be called 'advice' if it were), there is an 'expectation' that 'its recommendations on technologies will be universally accepted', and Rawlins warns that 'health professionals would be wise to record their reasons for non-compliance' with NICE guidelines in patients' medical records.

Rawlins' concerns appear eminently reasonable. It seems obvious that a good practitioner (even more so an 'excellent' one) will know what he or she is doing, and surely the sources of knowledge in clinical practice are the various forms of evidence available to the clinician. Analytically, a clinician unaware of the existing body of scientific research concerning the conditions he or she is treating is less well placed to understand those conditions than one in possession of this knowledge. Equally, the idea that unexplained variations in practice are undesirable is grounded in a widely held belief about rationality. If two people's conditions are the same, but I nonetheless treat them differently, then my behaviour seems to violate the basic rational requirement of consistency: treat like cases similarly. This idea is behind a popular view about good scientific practice, i.e. that properly scientific methods combine detailed observation with the rigorous application of deductive reasoning. If factors A, B and C give me grounds to infer X in one case, then the presence of the same factors should lead me to make the same inference in another case, and if they do not, then (in the absence of further explanation) my reasoning has been exposed as flawed. (If I say that I had a hunch that a different conclusion was appropriate, or that in my professional judgement they just 'felt' different, then – unless I can back this up with some clear, *observed* difference – I am likely to be condemned for being 'subjective', 'unscientific' and, by implication, irrational.) It is this same conception of rationality that in the moral sphere underlies our intuition that various forms of arbitrary discrimination are unacceptable. The concern that practices in the health service should be cost-effective also appears innocuous, and has been given an admirably clear defence by various health economists (most notably, Williams (1992, 1995), but see also my response to Williams (Loughlin M 1996b)).

Yet, if we give a little more critical attention to the concepts of knowledge, evidence, science and rationality, we soon see that the issues are not so straightforward. I noted earlier that certain assumptions may be implicit in a person's views about what features of the world *require* explanation, and what is to be treated as part of an uncontentious background. Clearly, Rawlins thinks that variation in clinical practice falls into the former category, requiring a special account, rather than viewing it as only to be expected, given the nature of the practice under consideration. Thus while Rawlins does not aim to rule out variation altogether (nor does he state unequivocally that it is a bad thing), there is a predisposition against it: rather like the presumption of innocence in law; in the case of variation, however, the presumption is to find it guilty in the absence of any arguments to the contrary. The onus is clearly assumed to be upon those who support a plurality of approaches to any given problem being employed at any given time to defend so (intuitively) suspect an idea. This is why the word 'variations' is usually preceded by some negative qualifying term such as 'inappropriate', 'unexplained' or 'unacceptable' (Rawlins 1999) and the image of a service in which practice is much more standardised than at present is presented as something of a utopian ideal. (That is to say, the existence of widespread variation in practice is presented as *cause for concern*, suggesting a gap between the way the service is now and the way it should be. A judgement of this sort logically implies a conception of the ideal with which to contrast reality and find it wanting, even though one readily admits that the gap between ideal and reality may never be eliminated entirely.)

The idea that rationality requires that we treat like cases similarly goes back at least as far as Aristotle's assertion (in the context of his discussion of justice) that we should treat equals equally, and unequals unequally (Aristotle, Thompson translator 1956). In fact it goes back even further than this, but the Aristotelian characterisation is useful for our present purposes, since it brings out the epistemological problems that arise when we attempt to apply this apparently straightforward principle. For the second part of the Aristotelian maxim, about treating unequals unequally, is just as important as the first. It is just as irrational to treat relevantly dissimilar cases in the same way as it is to treat relevantly similar cases differently. A problem arises when we consider how, in the first place, we identify *relevant* similarities and differences. Unfortunately, real situations do not come with labels: their equality (or lack thereof) is not stamped upon them for all to see. It is necessary for subjects to make decisions about which features of a situation to discount and which to emphasise when making judgements about whether or not a situation is of 'the same' type (therefore requiring 'the same' response) as another. No purely formal principle contains within itself the criteria for its proper application in practice. (Thus Aristotle notoriously thought that the differences between the people he called 'barbarians' and his fellow Greeks meant that there were no rational objections to the Greek practice of making their fellow human beings into slaves.) The gap between the general principle and the specifics of any given situation must, necessarily, be bridged by the interpretation of the agent facing that situation in practice. Individual judgement is therefore essential, and there will always be room for debate about whether the principle is being properly applied in a given case.

What follows from this? First of all, it is no longer so obvious what is meant by the claim that all decisions should be based on evidence. Like the claims that 'no-one is opposed to quality' and that rationality requires treating like cases alike, as a purely formal claim this appears uncontentious. However, since all reasoning requires making decisions about what to *count* as evidence in the first place, this claim cannot be used in support of any single conception of good scientific practice – and certainly not the deliberately simplistic deductivist account sketched above. No one today would seriously defend the idea that scientific reasoning is simply a matter of being aware of the evidence and drawing logical conclusions from it on the basis of deductive reasoning alone (see Miles *et al.* 1998). All credible positions in the philosophy of science (and I include among the credible theorists people as different as Popper and Feyerabend) accept that observation is a theory-laden exercise, that subjective judgements about the selection of the data to form the basis for conclusions are ineliminable, and that in all the most interesting and important areas of science the available data do not determine, deductively, any one theoretical position as *evidently* correct. No science (not even, it would appear, mathematics, and certainly not medicine) can purport to offer general conclusions which are *certain* and have concrete implications for *specific* cases. Individual judgement is not infallible, but nor can we do without it: to condemn it as 'subjective' in some reprehensible sense is to make scientific reasoning impossible (Loughlin AJ 1998, pp.95–121).

This suggests two related problems with regard to Rawlins' stance concerning variation. First, one might argue that, given the complex and diverse nature of human subjects, variation in the way they are treated is only to be expected, and it is the level of homogeneity in the treatment of NHS patients that requires explanation and should cause suspicion. The idea that patients can be reduced to sets of labels for conditions is part of a caricature of poor medical practice which it is doubtful that anyone would seriously attempt to defend. Each patient's condition is determined by a unique set of circumstances such that, the more direct acquaintance one has with the features of the person's particular circumstances that make him or her *different* from others with the same general type of problem, the more hope one has of actually *understanding* that person's problem. In an ideal world, the doctor would have much more time to become acquainted with each specific case, and it is by no means clear that this would tend to *standardise* practice: if anything, it would suggest more variation. The standardisation of practices is at least in part a response to economic constraints, not a reflection of some general principle that the more similarly you treat different cases, the more likely your treatment in each specific case is to be effective. In this context, viewing variation as something bad potentially suggests confusing economic considerations (such as the concern that efficient use be made of valuable time) with the desire to give each patient the sort of treatment appropriate to his or her specific case.

This is suggested further by Rawlins' failure to acknowledge openly a potential *conflict* between the different objectives of NICE. Rawlins typically equates the 'excellence' of a particular technology not only with its *clinical* but also with its *cost*-effectiveness. He notes that 'NICE will sometimes be forced to reject a particular technology' despite its effectiveness in a clinical context 'in the interests of the service as a whole' (Rawlins 1999, p.1082). In such a case, NICE would have to make a judgement that the benefits purchased for some patients would be outweighed by the sacrifices borne by others, given the financial cost of the technology and the limitations on NHS funding. In a display of word-play worthy of a politician or management specialist, Rawlins insists that this has nothing to do with cutting costs or 'rationing'. (Both his dictionary and his personal experience during the war tell him that 'rationing' is all about such activities as queueing for tins of spam.) Rather, it is about getting 'value for money', which is quite a different matter.

I fail to grasp the substantial difference in semantic content between the phrases 'controlling costs' and 'getting value for money'. If a technology serves its purpose very well, but is rejected because it is not 'value for money' (meaning, presumably, that its benefits do not justify its *cost*), it is nonsense to maintain that this decision has nothing to do with controlling costs. Whatever phrase we use, the substantial point remains that to treat both clinical and cost-effectiveness as dimensions of 'excellence' is to blur the obvious distinctions between the two. 'Excellence' and 'low costs' may go hand in hand in management theory, but in no other context would people make the mistake of equating them. Rawlins knows very well that the houses in his area which he would call 'excellent' are not likely also to be the cheapest. By and large, the more money you are prepared to pay, the more likely you are to be able to afford an 'excellent' property, and the smaller your budget, the less valuable a house you can afford. Similarly, in the context of the health service, the need to be cost-effective quite obviously places limits on the pursuit of 'clinical excellence'. To fudge this point is to disguise the fact that limitations upon cost affect the quality of care available to patients, and *not* by making it more 'excellent' (in any plausible sense of this word). We can only have an honest debate about rationing if we are willing to call it for what it is: if people in this country really are no longer willing to fund adequate public services out of taxation, then let them know what their decision means. The worst thing to do is to allow people to delude themselves that spending restrictions will in fact *improve* the 'quality' of the service.

In any case, when making judgements about 'value for money', even if we agree that the financial side of the equation is a quantifiable matter, the 'value' component to the calculation is riddled with the sort of controversies which preoccupy those who are prepared honestly to debate rationing. In deciding which treatments are worth funding, what conception of value will the decision-makers of NICE be employing? How do they defend it? Is it 'transparent', open to public debate? What if an individual has a conscientious disagreement about what is important? By what *right* will NICE (or CHI) impose its judgements upon dissenters? Does a background in science (or, come to that, moral philosophy) make you an expert on *what is important*? Does this notion make any sense? To function as rational beings we need to learn that others can, with good reason, disagree with us. This should be particularly obvious when it comes to questions of value. Rawlins says he hopes that his 'clinical colleagues' will 'accept', when their judgements about the value of funding certain treatments are overridden, that 'the Institute is committed to ensuring an equitable distribution of finite NHS resources'. Yet nowhere does Rawlins provide even an indication, let alone a detailed exposition and defence, of his specific conception of 'equity', so it is in no way clear why he thinks his fellow clinicians, or any other rational person whose interests may be affected by his decisions, should 'accept' the Institute's authority on such matters. It is one thing to accept that another person is *committed* to equity. It is another thing altogether to accept their right to pronounce authoritatively on what is equitable. If the only reason on offer is the brute fact of the NHS power structure, and NICE's position within it, then this hardly constitutes an *argument* in defence (or in favour) of that arrangement. Indeed, to admit this would be to admit that the position is in fact unarguable.

This brings us to the second problem with Rawlins' suspicion of variation. Many issues in clinical practice, not just those most directly and obviously concerned with value judgements, are highly contentious. To describe an issue as 'contentious' in an interesting sense is not merely to note the sheer possibility of disagreement: rather it is to note that there are issues such that, given the sum total of human knowledge at a given point in time, there is room for rational, informed persons to disagree, without this giving us cause to question the rationality of the parties in disagreement. Variation in practice is often a product of variation in judgement or interpretation of evidence. Rawlins accepts this, acknowledging that even clinical guidelines which are 'based on a rigorous and systematic review of all the relevant data must necessarily carry an element of judgement in their interpretation that may not be universally shared' (ibid., p.1081). However, he does not explain how this acknowledgement coheres with the decision to treat any one set of judgements as intellectually 'authoritative', simply because the persons making the judgements have the backing of the *political* authorities. To enshrine one set of judgements as 'authoritative' is to replace intellectual argument and debate with political authority. To describe that process as 'rational' or 'scientific' is to abuse these concepts.

The *rational* conclusion to draw is that we need to come to terms with human fallibility if we are to develop more realistic conceptions of scientific and professional practice (Popper 1989). Too many popular accounts of science take it as read that 'uncertainty' is a bad thing and 'evidence' is a good thing – the latter driving out the former like the white knight in pursuit of the dragon. Given this perception, the honest disagreement and debate which are the essence of a healthy scientific community become a cause for suspicion, suggesting that at least some members of that community do not 'know their stuff' and may, by implication, be incompetent. With the recognition that a degree of uncertainty is an essential feature of the human condition, come the virtues of humility and tolerance: one is able to be open to alternative approaches and realise that one's own assumptions and judgements are just one set among many. In the absence of any one certain method of discovering the truth, it is rational to tolerate a plurality of approaches: to refuse to do so is to close off potentially fruitful avenues of investigation *arbitrarily* (Feyerabend 1988). These points suggest it is folly to set up a single 'source of advice' as 'authoritative', however wise that source and however willing it is to change its mind over time. Charlton (1993) provides a more honest and intelligent picture of the reality of professional knowledge, arguing that the best hope for progress in science rests with the preservation of 'a democratic community of individuals, none of whom has the authority to dictate what is "truth"'. He adds that while some scientists 'may be more authoritative than others ... none has overall authority' and he suggests that if 'NHS management wishes to apply the fruits of science to medicine, then it should replicate its structure in something of the devolved, democratic, and peer-influenced nature of science' (ibid., p.100) (see also Chapter 2). In an environment where there is (rightly) no one dominant theory, variation in practice comes with the territory, and instead of lamenting it or trying to stamp it out, we need to explain its necessity and *its utility*. We do not eliminate human fallibility simply by calling some central source an 'authority', any more than we make practices 'excellent' by so labelling them.

Conclusion

In the absence of a much more detailed exposition and defence of the conceptual foundations of NICE and CHI, we have strong reason to question the claims made on behalf of these organisations. There are a number of serious problems with the very idea that a central body can legitimately pronounce authoritatively on good practice in the health service. Thus the claim that, by ensuring that centrally developed guidelines are widely followed, these organisations will facilitate the 'improvement' of practice must be treated with extreme scepticism. If the only backing for the claim to have 'authority' is the support of the powers that be, then such organisations represent a serious threat to academic freedom and scientific progress. The idea that their existence can serve the long-term interests of the populace at large must therefore also be questioned.

References

Al-Assaf AF & Schmele JA (ed.) (1993). *The textbook of total quality in healthcare.* St Lucie Press, Delray Beach, Florida, USA.

Aristotle. *Ethics* (JAK Thompson, translator, 1956). Penguin Books Ltd, Harmondsworth, Middlesex.

Berwick DM (1993). Continuous improvement as an ideal in health care. In *The textbook of total quality in healthcare* (ed. AF Al-Assaf & JA Schmele), pp.31–9. St Lucie Press, Delray Beach, Florida, USA.

Charlton BG (1993). Management of science. *Lancet* **342,** 99–100.

Curtis K (1993). Total quality and management philosophies. In *The textbook of total quality in healthcare* (ed. AF Al-Assaf & JA Schmele), pp.191–205. St Lucie Press, Delray Beach, Florida, USA.

Feyerabend P (1988). *Against method.* Verso Books, London.

Heginbotham C (1994). Management worries [Letter to the editor]. *Health Care Analysis* **2,** 270.

[IHSM] The Institute of Health Services Management (1993). *Future health care options, final report.* IHSM, London.

Joss, R & Kogan M (1995). *Advancing quality: total quality management in the National Health Service.* Open University Press, Buckingham.

Laffel G & Blumenthal D (1993). The case for using industrial quality management science in health care organisations. In *The textbook of total quality in healthcare* (ed. AF Al-Assaf & JA Schmele), pp.40–50. St Lucie Press, Delray Beach, Florida, USA.

Liddle A (1992). Health gain. Proceedings from The Standing Conference, Norwich 23–24 July. *Health Gain* **92.**

Loughlin AJ (1998). *Alienation and value-neutrality.* Ashgate Publishing Ltd, Aldershot.

Loughlin M (1993). The illusion of quality. *Health Care Analysis* **1,** 69–73.

Loughlin M (1994a). Behind the wall paper. *Health Care Analysis* **2,** 47–53.

Loughlin M (1994b). The poverty of management. *Health Care Analysis* **2,** 135–9.

Loughlin M (1996a). The language of quality. *Journal of Evaluation in Clinical Practice* **2,** 87–95.

Loughlin M (1996b). Rationing, barbarity and the economist's perspective. *Health Care Analysis* **4,** 146–56.

Merry M (1993). Total quality management for physicians: translating the new paradigm. In *The textbook of total quality in healthcare* (ed. AF Al-Assaf & JA Schmele), pp.51–9. St Lucie Press, Delray Beach, Florida, USA.

Miles A, Bentley P, Grey J & Polychronis A (1995). Purchasing quality in clinical practice: what on Earth do we mean? *Journal of Evaluation in Clinical Practice* **1,** 87–95.

Miles A, Bentley P, Polychronis A, Grey J & Price N (1998). Recent progress in health services research: on the need for evidence-based debate. *Journal of Evaluation in Clinical Practice* **4,** 257–65.

Peters DA (1992). A new look for quality in home care. *Journal of Nursing Administration* **22,** 21–6.

Popper K (1989). *Objective knowledge: an evolutionary approach.* Clarendon Press, Oxford.

Rawlins (1999). In pursuit of quality: the National Institute for Clinical Excellence. *The Lancet* **353,** 1079–82.

Stevenson CL (1944). *Ethics and Language.* Gollancz, London.

Wall A (1994). Behind the wallpaper: a rejoinder. *Health Care Analysis* **2,** 317–18.

Williams A (1992). Cost-effectiveness analysis: is it ethical? *Journal of Medical Ethics* **18,** 7–11.

Williams A (1995). Economics, QALYs and medical ethics – a health economist's perspective. *Health Care Analysis* **3,** 221–6.

Chapter 2

The new management of scientific knowledge in medicine: a change of direction with profound implications

Bruce G Charlton

Introduction

In 1993 I published a *Lancet* Viewpoint entitled 'Management of science' in which I pointed out that purchasing managers in the National Health Service had begun implementing very precise contracts which controlled detailed aspects of clinical practice (Charlton 1993). For instance, it became mandatory to specify protocols for beta-blocker and aspirin treatment following myocardial infarction, and for prescription of benzodiazepines, antidepressants and other psychotropic drugs, and for aspects of skin cancer management. The justification for these blanket recommendations was that these interventions were 'scientifically' proven to be effective across the board in almost every clinical circumstance – at least according to the NHS Management Executive's interpretation of the results of large randomised trials (although expert clinicians may frequently have disagreed; see, for example, Julian (1995)).

But the fundamental problem was structural: the Government was creating a managerial structure that separated the power to influence treatment from clinical responsibility for the consequences of that treatment. For example, managers were claiming the right to determine the nature of a drug prescription, while doctors remained both morally and legally responsible for the outcome. This seemed self-evidently unethical, and placed doctors in the impossible position of being vulnerable to sacking if they were disobedient, and to malpractice suits if they obeyed. The system was also open to corruption, since political influence could be brought to bear on managers, tending to generate protocols using criteria dictated by expediency rather than by effectiveness. For example, the call for specified protocols on psychotropic drugs was unsupported by any rational consensus on what such protocols should contain, and the instructions concerning 'skin' cancer (and the failure to differentiate between basal cell, squamous cell and melanomatous malignancies) seemed more justified by the immediate demands of public relations than by any body of solid scientific evidence.

As things turn out, I had underestimated the seriousness of this kind of threat to clinical practice, and my article unfortunately proved to be prophetic of a trend which has culminated in the creation of the National Institute for Clinical Excellence (NICE) and the Commission for Health Improvement (CHI). The management of science in medicine is now established by statute, and – even worse – the criteria of effectiveness have been conflated with economic considerations of 'cost-effectiveness'. The stage is set for clinical science to be steamrollered by the demands of power politics.

The evidential basis of NICE guidelines – the number-crunching commissars

NICE and CHI are organised in the form of a statutory arm of the government bureaucracy, as special health authorities with powers intended to influence the clinical practice of doctors and other health workers. The credibility of NICE and CHI depends crucially upon the claim that NICE guidelines will be objectively valid – based on appropriate evidence, properly interpreted, rationally argued and intellectually compelling. Only if this is true will NICE guidelines possess the necessary legitimacy such that failure to adhere to them would reasonably be interpretable as negligence. But if NICE guidelines are seen to be partisan, irrational, scientifically unconvincing or politically driven, then they will amount to little more than government propaganda backed up with a big stick.

NICE advertises itself as the application of rational and scientific management to medical practice. In particular, the claimed intellectual credibility of NICE and CHI derives from a whole raft of data-driven and statistically based academic disciplines which have become dominant in the past decade. These include health economics, epidemiology, evidence-based medicine (EBM) and related areas of research concerning clinical effectiveness, meta-analysis, unexplained variations in practice, guidelines, and so on. All of these activities in the UK (activities which I term 'Infostat' – see below) have been created, sustained and directed largely by Department of Health funding. In return for this funding, the practitioners of these arts have performed (sometimes unwittingly) a managerial role – having the *de facto* function of *commissars* for Government and the NHS management (*q.v.* the role of intellectuals in Stalinist USSR (Joravsky 1970)). Infostat technicians can be seen as having prepared public and professional opinion for the emergence of NICE and CHI and the statutory government regulation of clinical practice (Charlton & Miles 1998).

NICE has no extraordinary access to evidence, nor does it have any extraordinary technique for analysing evidence, nor are its decision-making processes anything extraordinary for a special health authority. There is therefore no reason to assume that NICE will perform any better than any other government bureaucracy when it comes to providing objective, rational and independent guidance. Given these facts, the statutory powers of NICE and CHI seem implicitly to assert that there can be *no genuine or principled uncertainty* about the proper nature of guidelines, since, if there were, then the *coercive* imposition of guidelines would not be justifiable.

Problems with randomised controlled trials

For NICE guidelines to be credible, it ought to be clear to any informed and disinterested party that optimal clinical practice – in each *specific instance* for which guidelines are used – is known, and can be stated clearly and exactly in the form of usable guidelines. Presumably, this implies that randomised controlled trials (RCTs) are intended to be the main source of evidence for NICE, since it is a commonly held belief among the clinically ignorant and epidemiologically unsophisticated that the RCT method is capable of providing precise and unambiguous ('gold standard') guidance for clinical practice (see, for example, Sackett *et al.* (1985) or, indeed, any publication you care to select from the EBM movement, *Effectiveness Bulletins* or the Cochrane Collaboration).

Unfortunately for NICE, RCTs cannot provide precise and unambiguous guidance for clinical practice (Feinstein 1995; Charlton 1996a, 1996b, 1997; Goodman 1998, 1999). The increasing proliferation of 'evidence-based' clinical advice and guidance purports to be objectively valid according to the notion that large randomised trials provide the best guidance for clinical practice. But in reality these RCT-based guidelines have proved to be just as unreliable as any other sources of advice. This was inevitable, since most randomised trials are conducted on unrepresentative populations of heterogeneous subjects and employ suboptimal levels of experimental control. The interpretation of such trials is usually far from straightforward and may be impossible (Goodman 1999).

Many bio-statisticians hoped that meta-analysis would solve this problem and provide a method for objective interpretation. But this was also a delusion, since an accumulation of inadequate data simply makes a bigger pile of inadequate data, and the statistical averaging of different trials performed in different places by different people for different purposes merely generates a meaningless statistical artefact. To put it bluntly, meta-analysis is a logically incoherent technique of zero scientific credibility (Feinstein 1995; Charlton 1996b). It is embarrassing for those who under-stand statistics and clinical medicine to contemplate the innocent enthusiasm of its supporters, and profoundly worrying that their armour-plated credulity has become the orthodoxy among politicians and managers. Meta-analysis never was adequate or appropriate to the task of decision-making and arbitration wished upon it by the protagonists of EBM; and even within its limited statistical purview, the disagreements between supposedly 'objective' meta-analyses have devastated the credibility of the method (Bailar 1997).

The failure of RCTs and meta-analysis to deliver objective and authoritative guidelines means that NICE recommendations will inevitably suffer from the same lack of intellectual credibility that afflicts the many other sources of supposedly definitive guidelines emanating from the DoH-sponsored guidelines industry (NHS Centre for Reviews and Dissemination, Cochrane Collaboration, etc.). NICE guidelines will differ from existing sources of medical advice only because they will be mandatory and enforced on doctors by sanctions.

How science works

Since science is the major source of 'reliable knowledge' (Ziman 1978), and that is what NICE is claiming to base its guidelines upon, one approach to evaluating the decision-making processes of NICE is to compare the workings of NICE with the workings of science (Hull 1988).

In scientific practice, rival theories are proposed by the many individuals and groups working in a field of endeavour. Alternative observations, experiments and interpretations emerge from different directions. Disagreement and dissent (whether over fundamentals or over minutiae) is the normal state of affairs in any *active* subject within science. Yet as well as being a locus of disagreement and dissent, science has been characterised by its being progressive, an accumulation of tested knowledge. Despite disagreement, some scientific theories are accepted and built upon, while others (indeed, typically the bulk of scientific work produced) are either ignored or rejected. Who decides what is ignored and what is incorporated? Who winnows the wheat from the chaff?

The answer is that no specific person or group decides, but that scientific 'truth' *emerges* in the working practices of other scientists who are active in the field (Hull 1988). The ultimate judge of scientific validity is to have your work *used* by other scientists in their work, and the ultimate prestige is to be acknowledged as the originator of work that is being so used. And it is this testing by use, by others, in practice and in competition with other theories, which stands at the root of the objectivity of science.

For example, there was no central committee or individual who decided that Crick and Watson's double helix structure for DNA was correct, and that this 'true' theory should be imposed upon other biologists (Judson 1979). Rather, the structure was used by other biochemists in their own researches. In a nutshell, when it was assumed that the double helix structure *was* true, scientists were able to predict observations, perform experiments and make manipulations that *worked*. The truth of the structure was not therefore decided, it emerged in practice.

Not every biologist agreed that Crick and Watson were correct, and nobody tried to coerce these people into adopting the double helix theory. However, over time, it emerged that those who disagreed were not able to 'knock down' the double helix structure to the satisfaction of other workers in the field, nor were they able to produce a similarly powerful explanatory alternative structure to the double helix (Judson 1979). The dissenters were starved of status and influence, and have largely disappeared from the scene by a process akin to selection, whereby the pro-double helix scientists 'reproduced' and left scientific descendants, while the anti-double helix scientists failed to reproduce and became (more or less) extinct (Hull 1988).

This is the kind of winnowing process that gives scientific knowledge its validity; the propositions of valid science have been tested by use. Validity is therefore pragmatic with respect to the *natural world*. If a scientific theory stops working when trying to explain and predict the natural world, or if something better comes along, then the scientists who advocate their theory will find that their work, hence their careers, are stalled (so long as they are honest, and do not fabricate or misrepresent their results – and science depends absolutely upon the honesty of its practitioners (Bronowski 1975)). The situation then becomes ripe for the death of that theory and its replacement.

Scientific knowledge is therefore both tentative (subject to revision) and also objective (in the sense that the decision about validity is made by the community of active scientists using natural world criteria – and not by the person who devises the theory, nor by any specific minority group) (see Hull 1988).

Summary of the nature of scientific decision-making

- The cumulative and progressive nature of science depends on a type of social structure for testing theories in practice against the natural world.
- When science is working properly, arbitration concerning the 'truth' of scientific theories depends upon active scientific practitioners who *use* that theory in their work.
- In science power is dispersed among practitioners. Truth *emerges* from the social structure of science in a way that is beyond the power of any individual or group to determine.
- The personal motivation driving the system of arbitration is the personal interest of the arbitrators. In science the power to arbitrate goes with personal responsibility for the consequences. To 'believe' in a theory is equivalent to staking one's own practice (hence reputation, hence career) on its validity.
- Scientific 'truth' is therefore something that is tested against the constraints of the natural world in the practice of its active workers. The bottom line is the test of the natural world.
- The ultimate scientific sanction to enforce a theory upon the practitioner is whether it is consistent with observed phenomena – the sanction is that the constraints of the natural world will 'sabotage' the work of a scientist who uses false theories.

The social structure of NICE and CHI

It has been necessary to spell out the way in which science works, in particular how decision-making depends upon the social structure of science, in order to contrast this with the social structure of NICE and CHI. Here are a few of the differences:

- NICE and CHI are part of the executive arm of Government, performing roles established by statute.
- NICE and CHI are near the apex of a top-down managerial hierarchy in which the upper echelons audit and control the lower ones. This means that non-practitioners make decisions and enforce those decisions upon practitioners.
- Power to judge scientific theories in NICE and CHI is centralised and concentrated in the hands of the few who give orders to be acted upon by the many.

- The personal motivation driving the system of arbitration comprises the usual incentives of officials working in a bureaucratic structure. The career and status of a managerial arbitrator do not depend primarily upon getting the scientific decisions correct; rather, career and status depend primarily upon satisfying the internal demands of the system. The real world consequences of the theory impinge on the practitioners, not the managers.
- NICE redefines 'science' as being whatever the outcomes of its deliberations are. Since decisions are in the hands of the few, this decision-making process is readily corrupted by political expediency, external pressure, or self-interest. The bottom line is keeping the boss happy.
- The sanctions imposing the views of NICE derive from the world of politics, not from the natural world.

Managerial take-over of the NHS

From administration to management

The creation of NICE and CHI can be interpreted as the most recent and aggressive expression of a managerial take-over of the NHS which has been going on for several decades. Managers can be defined as staff concerned with second-order activities – such as policy, finance and organisational planning – as contrasted with practitioners who perform the core tasks of the organisation. As Simon Jenkins (1995) has put it: 'The achievement of the Thatcher reforms was to make [NHS] management centralised and supreme'.

One of the most important changes since the NHS began was the transformation of administrators to managers. There was more to this than a mere change in name – it represented a change in philosophy. Administrators are an unavoidable element in large organisations of any size – managers are an optional extra. Health service *administrators* had the secondary (albeit vital) role of running the organisational side of the NHS. Their job was to make a framework for professionals to exercise judgement within; they sought to implement the regulations and 'oil the wheels'. Broadly, they aspired to the civil service ideal of impartiality and advice rather than control.

But the role of managers is rather different. Managers are primary. They do not just implement regulations, they make regulations; they do not just make a framework for judgement, they dictate the processes and outcomes of judgement; they are committed, not impartial; they give orders rather than offering advice; they commission new wheels rather than oiling existing ones. In this sense, NICE is managerial, rather than administrative – it is designed to dominate professionals, not to assist them.

Central control versus devolved autonomy

In the old NHS, authority was assumed to lie with the clinical professionals by virtue of their skills, traditions and patient contact, so that once the organisational structure was established, detailed policy (such as it was) was to a great extent implicit and *emergent* from the interactions of clinicians, administrators and politicians. That is to say, policy was bottom-up rather than top-down. The 1980s, by contrast, saw a trend towards *dirigisme* with a massive expansion in the powers of central government (Klein 1989; Jenkins 1995). The NHS 'reforms' brought more government – albeit rationalised as serving the long-term goal of *less* government. This politicisation of the NHS ushered in a new era in which the service was to be driven from above by radical ideas emanating in broad outline from the cabinet and its policy think-tanks, and implemented in detail by an executive management, empowered to impose these upon an unwilling and resistant professional and ancillary workforce.

The first wave of general managers were therefore pretty much tools of government policy. They were accountancy-oriented hit men, focused almost exclusively on financial reorganisation: implementing cuts in funding, introducing 'efficiency'-enhancing measures (privatisation, contracting-out) and, in general, having an attitude to the NHS that reflected the Prime Minister of the day. This period established the dominance of the way of thinking that sees the NHS primarily in generic organisational and economic terms – and not as specifically a *health* service.

Initially, at least, managers were engaged upon managing down to the level of clinical consultation, but not beyond. The interface between the public and the health professional remained out of bounds. Clinical decision-making was left largely independent and untouched by direct mechanisms, although it was influenced by organisational and resource constraints and, in turn, influenced them. Since that time, a path has been followed that establishes financial control by encroaching on clinical independence and seeking increasing control of decision-making. Over the years the managerial agenda has therefore moved towards direct influence of decision-making processes in the clinical consultation, and towards pre-determination of the possible outcomes of doctor-patient interactions.

Dominance of general management

In an important sense, the single unifying thrust of recent NHS reforms has been the transfer of power from health professionals – principally doctors – to a new class of employees: general managers (Charlton 1993). 'General management', as it was called by the Griffiths report (1983), gets its title from the intellectual rationale which lies behind the decision to put managers in charge of the NHS. It was asserted that the skills of management were *generic*, i.e. non-specific, transferable between different situations, and applicable equally to private sector retail and public sector service organisations, and to all types of social function.

General management was the answer to what Griffiths saw as the main problem of the NHS, that exactly nobody was 'in charge'. In actuality this matter of nobody being 'in charge' of the NHS was only partly accidental and regrettable. It was also partly an inevitable and desirable aspect of a collegial and democratic organisation based upon the work of skilled professionals dealing with clients whose views must also be taken into account. The accidental and regrettable aspects of nobody being in charge were largely a consequence of the previous set of Conservative NHS reforms in 1974, which – in seeking to diminish the power of doctors, and achieve a broad representation of interest groups – had succeeded only in creating a gridlock at the level of policy and planning (Klein 1989). The log-jam certainly needed unblocking, and personally responsible, dynamic general managers were a good swap for sclerotic and unaccountable committees. The massively increased programme of hospital-building in the past decade is evidence of the consequential improvement in executive planning.

However, the implementers of the Griffiths report seem not to have appreciated that an organisation depending upon the skills of autonomous health professionals will not function properly if it has imposed on it a hierarchical, line-managed, heavily regulated structure imported from businesses based on simpler and more routine activities, and lacking the necessary personal relationship between providers and clients which characterises medicine. Since 1983, it has been the long-term intention that the *primary focus* of NHS activity was to be the management of the organisation, rather than the personal interactions between clinicians and patients. From this it followed that managers were obviously the best people to run the show. The essence of the successive waves of NHS reforms has been to make possible this managerial take-over.

General management was *imposed* upon the NHS (Klein 1989; Jenkins 1995). Management did not evolve organically in response to the demands of the system, but was grafted onto the existing system because this was felt to be what the system needed (or, if not needed, then deserved). The intention was that general management transplanted from the private sector would take over from the clinical professionals in a kind of 'graft versus host' reaction.

The enhanced role of policy and planning in NHS affairs

There is more to general management than a transfer of power from clinicians to managers. Alongside, there has been a trend towards explicit, top-down policy and planning. Power is now more concentrated at upper levels and in managerial chains of command, and clinical interactions are increasingly constrained: doctors have less autonomy and patients have less influence over the clinical consultation despite the political rhetoric that they should have more.

The superficial aspects of this dominance of policy and planning are familiar: they comprise the whole bogus rhetoric of mission statements, aims and objectives, targets, charters, standards, guidelines, protocols, publicity, public relations and packaging – the rising tide of 'bullshit and bollocks', as the playwright Alan Plater has vividly and succinctly described it.

But the deeper role of policy has acted synergistically to increase the rate of policy *change* in the NHS. Clinical practice is, of course, familiar with change – having re-invented itself several times in response to therapeutic innovation over the past 60 years (Le Fanu 1999). And such clinical change leads to policy changes, but by an indirect, implicit, bottom-up route. At present, however, there is almost an *expectation* of rapid changes in policy at the large scale or 'macro'-level. This is apparently what 'dynamic' management is all about – making structural alterations ('permanent revolution' as Mao Tse Tung put it, or 'thriving on chaos', as management guru Tom Peters (1989) puts it). Changing organisational structures is how managers make their reputations and maintain their power (Charlton 1995).

High-level strategy synergises with low-level shell-shock to entrench managerial dominance; and only those whose heads are above the fray are able to safeguard their own interests. The managerial literature therefore, unsurprisingly, regards changing an organisation as admirable in itself. We are all familiar with the phoney nomenclature whereby every threat is seen as a 'challenge', every disaster seen as presenting an 'opportunity'. All this translates as organisational change creating an increased scope for shrewd managers to attain rapid career enhancement. Meanwhile, clinicians and other practitioners are kept busier than ever on 'fire-fighting' tasks: implementing reforms, increasing productivity, negotiating rationing of services and generally squaring the circle where central planning meets market forces and patient demands.

Macro-strategy leads to micro-tactics. Frequent shifts in overall direction at high levels create endemic insecurity at the lower levels (redeployment, redundancy, retraining). Chaos translates into increased uncertainty at the level of personal goals and interactions, with an accompanying narrowing of perspective and shortening of time horizons. The contemporary NHS is characterised by an official versus unofficial schism – far-sightedness and bold ambition among the planners, with a survivalist mentality among the planned.

The chaos game is one that only managers and politicians can 'thrive' on: professionals and patients are the losers. Those aspects of the NHS reforms destructive of the provision of clinical services are often excused or minimised by policy-minded commentators, on the basis that 'at least' the reforms initiated *change*. This perspective presumes that the NHS was so bad that change could only be for the better, and contrasts sharply with the perspective of practitioners and patients who tend to be impressed only by improvements, rather than by change *per se*. The difference is that clinicians and clients seek evidence that change will be positive, otherwise they support the *status quo*; managers seek a system where change *is* the *status quo*. All groups are, of course, self-interested. But the self-interest of practitioners is closer to the needs of the public – not least because individual patients can exert direct influence by means of the personal relationship that is the clinical consultation.

The problem of legitimacy

General management was created to be 'in charge' of the NHS, and was imposed upon the organisation following an era from 1974 when *nobody* was in charge of the

NHS (the health service was supposed to be run by consensus, but in action was blocked by huge committees paralysed by vetoes (Klein 1989)). However, power in the NHS is importantly conditional upon consent and cannot be wielded unilaterally. To be effective, power must be perceived as legitimate. And legitimacy can seldom be conferred by diktat; the holders of power must be seen as entitled in some way, or else resistance will be excessive.

The legitimacy of general management was initially seriously lacking. Indeed, how could matters be otherwise given the lack of relevant knowledge and experience of most of the newly appointed managers? Aside from some NHS administrators who underwent the transition to manager, the early cohorts of general managers were pretty much whisked up out of thin air, under the above-mentioned belief that management skills were generic. This view was not widely shared *within* the health service, where it was assumed that running a military barracks, a sweet factory and a hospital presented significantly different challenges. Nonetheless, managers were bought in from the military and the private sectors, although the salaries and conditions on offer from the NHS were insufficiently attractive to get the best personnel, and the early cohorts of managers were considered to be insufficiently competent.

Managerial influence on the NHS was initially dependent upon various crude threats (resource cutbacks, closures, sacking, etc.) and the personal qualities of the manager. Probably the most effective managers were those who combined common sense and force of character. Since managerial authority was not backed up by any convincing expertise, and because solidarity among managers was undermined by short-term contracts and competition, there was a desperate search for a *technique* of management that would reliably impress clinicians and politicians alike, between whom managers were uncomfortably sandwiched in the NHS hierarchy. Rationalist management by 'Infostat' methods came along just in the nick of time. 'Infostat' is my term for the use of information technology and statistics to support and legitimate managerial decision-making (see below).

Outwitting the clinicians

So, from 1983 there has been a frantic scramble to plaster a veneer of reasonableness over the *fait accompli* of the managerial take-over of the NHS. There was a dual purpose: underwriting managerial legitimacy and undermining clinical legitimacy. Managers seized upon 'Infostat' techniques as the ideal tool for creating the authority necessary to perform their appointed role.

Clinicians are a problem. Not only are they frequently confident and articulate individuals prepared to argue their corner, but they have also traditionally been able to claim a special legitimacy for their views based upon experience, expertise and direct personal contact with patients, and this legitimacy has been supported by a broad public consensus. However, the clinical databases stored in the heads of doctors are jealously guarded and may be subjectively interpreted to benefit clinical interests. Managers can only log into them via the doctor, and since doctors are frequently the major obstacle to NHS management attaining its objectives, it was important for managers dedicated to gaining ascendancy over clinicians to denigrate clinical experience and open up direct access to alternative sources of data.

The lack of direct contact between patients and managers is, on the face of it, a great and apparently fatal disadvantage to their competence and credibility in assuming the mantle of advocates of public health. Infostat techniques can be seen as a response to this crucial deficiency, in that they aggrandise the significance of the large data base, denigrate the value of personal contact with patients (too 'anecdotal' and 'subjective'), and misrepresent the scope of statistical analysis as being the best and proper procedure for managerial decision-making (Charlton 1996b, 1997). Managers have embarked upon the collection and interpretation of large data bases in the knowledge that such sources of information are either unavailable to clinicians or else too inaccessible and unwieldy for busy doctors to interpret.

Much of the increased emphasis on explicit information and statistical analysis as tools of NHS policy can be seen as a rhetorical strategy with which to over-ride the claims of clinical professionals to a unique understanding of health issues. Increasingly, clinical training, experience and patient contact are derided as subjective, and marginalised as anecdotal compared with the awesome weight of 'comprehensive' health service data, and the dazzling power of 'objective' statistical analysis (see Miles *et al.* 1997, 1998). Whatever is not large scale, numerical and statistically processed, is seen as inadmissible evidence. And politicians and management have – through DoH funding of Infostat technologists – ensured that they have a virtual monopoly of such evidence and major influence over its interpretation and dissemination.

The scope and nature of Infostat technologies

'Infostat' is a neologism coined to describe managerial technologies which employ 'info'(-rmation) and subject it to 'stat'(-istical) analysis to support decision-making.

Infostat requires large quantities of data for it to be a plausible reflection of health service activity and to produce summary averages of impressive statistical precision. Its introduction has therefore been inextricably linked with demands for more information on more aspects of NHS activity. Insofar as Infostat is designed to legitimate the control of clinical interactions, this requires a greatly increased amount of data collection about clinical affairs. This managerial drive is what lies behind calls for 'accountability', 'transparency' and 'explicitness' in clinical decisions (Charlton 1999).

Such demands for information are neither driven by a clinical need, nor by reasons of organisational effectiveness or efficiency (although these goals may be used to excuse the demands for more data). Instead, the true drive behind increased information collection is the *managerial* need for more numerical data in relation to the activity of employees, so that employee activity can be more easily monitored and controlled.

Because data are used rhetorically, quantity of data is much more important than its quality. Indeed politicians and managers are almost indifferent to the *real* quality of data, and academic criticisms of validity, sampling and statistical appropriateness are like water off a duck's back, as it were, since they are entirely subsidiary to the managerial process. Technical criticisms may provide a focus for dissent, but do not affect the steady onward implementation of Infostat. The goal of managerial data collection is not so much a matter of *discovering* ways of legitimately reducing clinical activities to numerical data, but of the *necessity* for using numerical data to describe clinical activities. So long as the data have some kind of face validity or superficial plausibility – that is all that is required.

Hence at every level of the NHS an increased proportion of resources (personnel, time, effort, software, hardware) are now devoted to routine information collection and processing – and the trend continues unchecked. And all these newly available data are potentially available to be fed into Infostat mechanisms and used to support management decisions. Because, even though policy is not actually *dictated* by the outcomes of data collection and analysis, access to such accumulations of data is assumed to be a *pre-requisite* of competence to determine policy. In this game, statistics always trumps direct personal experience to the point that people are no longer supposed to act upon the evidence of their senses (Miles *et al.* 1998).

Pure statistical analysis is a neutral activity which does not make causal suppositions – ideally, it simply *clarifies* what was already there. But the major pitfalls of statistics arise when it comes to attaching real world entities to mathematical symbols and making statistical manipulations without regard for the relevant causal processes. There is almost unlimited scope for statistical malpractice in health service management because Infostat is apparently applicable to *any* problem so long as enough data can somehow be expressed quantitatively (Charlton 1997). Statistically precise measurement without an understanding of what the numbers represent is a snare to the incautious – and a constant temptation to the unscrupulous – because numerical exactitude is so often mistaken for understanding.

Modern NHS management operates on the basis that bad data are assumed to be better than no data at all: from the perspective of someone wishing to use statistics as a cosh to stun the clinical opposition, this is quite correct. But from the perspective of someone actually trying to run a good health service, then bad data generate wrong answers. The watchword, as always, is GIGO – 'garbage in, garbage out'. No matter how high-powered the statistics, conclusions cannot be stronger than the validity and representativeness of the data base from which they were generated.

The policy sausage-machine

NHS management is trying to create the illusion of a policy sausage-machine. The NHS sausage machine is fed on numerical data and disgorges rational policies. No thinking is necessary – all is pre-determined by objective information and statistics. Raw data are collected and loaded into a funnel at the top of NICE; the handle is turned; inputted information is ground up, mixed and segmented by statistical engines; and clinical guidelines are emitted in discrete but linked gobbets. NICE is portrayed as merely a *mechanism* for generating rational policies; CHI as merely a mechanism for monitoring and ensuring the implementation of these rational policies.

Of course it is all an illusion. The sausage machine is designed by politicians and operated by managers. Data input is selective, analysis is selective, and implementation is selective. The numerous political pressures and managerial judgements are shielded from critique by an elaborate facade of pseudo-evidence and quasi-mathematical impartiality. The official propaganda for NICE denies the massive role of arbitrary opinion and interest involved in deciding what *ought* to be done, and concentrates all its efforts on making people do it.

And what of doctors and the other clinicians and practitioners? The role of doctors is equivalent to stacking supermarket shelves and manning the checkouts – merely a question of receiving and distributing the sausages. The doctor's job is to be an obedient, receptive functionary, strictly following protocols; all significant decisions about the nature, content and range of sausages are made elsewhere and by other people. Miles *et al.* (2000a, 2000b) have recently lamented this process as the conversion of doctors as professionals to doctors as technicians.

Although much is made of 'public accountability' nowadays, the patient's job is merely to choose from the range of goods on display (sausages will, of course, be brightly packaged, and each will have a 'quality assurance' stamp[1]). The individual patient's interaction with the policy sausage machine cannot significantly influence clinical processes and outcomes. Personal relationships to the sausage sales assistants – I mean doctors – will be at the level of a fast food outlet: compulsorily cheerful, utterly stereotyped. The doctor is not allowed to take notice of individual patients' needs, wants and preferences – the doctor can only stick to procedure and act within a prescribed, pre-determined and limited range of responses.

NICE and CHI are our first taste of a world in which politicians and health service managers think they know *exactly* what doctors ought to be doing (after all, the Infostat commissars have analysed the data and told them *exactly* – to the third decimal place – what doctors ought to be doing). The obstacle that politicians and managers perceive in the path of optimal health care is that doctors will not always do what they are told. The medical profession is too strong. The only sensible solution is therefore to destroy the medical profession and *force* doctors (or if they still refuse, somebody else) to follow instructions.[2] By this account of clinical practice the doctor's role in the health service is not to exercise autonomous judgement: it is simply to *obey* guidelines.

This explains why doctors are – at the time of writing, and according to the Prime Minister's opening speech at the 1999 Labour Party conference – officially Public Enemy Number One. Doctors are to the present Government what the coal-miners were to Mrs Thatcher's Government – the symbolic group who stand in the path of the untrammelled will of the state, and whose power and credibility must be broken. In this sausage machine world, doctors are not an *answer* to the problem of providing health services; doctors themselves are the problem.

Doctors are no longer a group of people who in their practice actually *embody* the health service – rather they are merely one of several groups of people whose job it

---

1   The term 'NICE-approved' is already in use.
2   Witness the rise of the nurse practitioner and hospital pharmacist.

is to *deliver* health services. The actual nature of clinical service is no longer to be under the control of doctors, never mind patients, but will be decided by politicians and managers – allegedly on the basis of ever-increasing quantities of information and statistics. Who could argue with that?

The demand for Infostat

Why did the NHS end up on the path to this nightmare parody of a one-stop superstore? The most plausible answer is that present policies arose incrementally but inexorably from the initial decision to impose general management on the NHS: from the decision that the NHS must have a centralised leadership and hierarchical management in order that it be controllable by the Government.

Many of the newly appointed general managers of the 1980s were inexperienced, inexpert, unconfident and overwhelmed by the grandiose (and often impossible) tasks handed down to them from above. Even worse, managers found themselves blocked and intimidated by the self-confidence (and arrogance) of clinicians from below. Most managers came and went swiftly on their well-paid but short-term contracts. The unscrupulous among them achieved success as hit-and-run merchants – making a name with a new logo and letterhead, then up the ladder before anything could go wrong. Locations and roles changed so frequently that specific local knowledge of health and personnel had no time to develop. In other words, health service managers found themselves in a position analogous to Machiavelli's Prince to whom that infamous book of advice on manipulation and survival was addressed (Machiavelli, Marriott translator 1992).

In the words of the political philosopher Michael Oakeshott (1962):

*'Machiavelli wrote for the **new** prince of his day who brought to his task only the qualities that had enabled him to gain political power. Lacking education (except in the habits of ambition), and requiring some short cut to the appearance of education, he required a crib. The project of Machiavelli was, then, to provide a crib to politics, a political training in default of a political education, a technique for the ruler who had no tradition.'*

Infostat technologies have provided exactly the 'crib' that general management needed. In a real sense, general management was neither personally nor professionally competent to do the job it was given. Yet the job had to be done somehow – the BMW needs replacing, school fees escalate, mortgages must be paid. Managers needed a plausible rationale for their decisions and arguments to back them up. Such arguments must be of a sort designed if not to *convince* clinicians, then at least to neutralise, bamboozle, side-step or overwhelm clinical opposition. The ideal of Infostat is not to out-argue opposing viewpoints by decisive logical or scientific evidence, but instead to *bury* them under a sheer mass of *soi-disant* evidence.

In this managerial model, everything hinges upon gaining legitimacy for the Infostat crib. Infostat purports to capture the essence of what clinical practice ought to be. If it did, in fact, do so, then coercive managerial dominance over the consultation would be justifiable and probably desirable. If it does not – and the Infostat crib is merely a more or less plausible technical trick – then the NICE claim for legitimacy in controlling the doctor–patient interaction is exploded.

NICE as 'cargo-cult' science

Infostat bears some resemblance to science. But the Infostat technologies which led up to the creation of NICE are actually an example of what Richard Feynman (1986) called 'cargo-cult' science: an activity presenting the facade of science but without the substance. Feynman described how remote and undeveloped South Seas islands briefly enjoyed prosperity when used as US air bases during World War II. When peace came, the air force left, and with it the prosperity. On the islands quasi-religions developed with the goal of attracting cargo-bearing aeroplanes to return and restore the golden age. These cults took the trappings of a technological culture – runways, marker flares, control towers, headphones, aerials – but all constructed from wood and stone technology. Everything was assembled in the proper way, the appearance of everything seemed just about right, the people went through the right motions … but the planes never landed.

By analogy, Infostat has many of the trappings of science – researchers, data collection, statistics, large grants, and publications. Its practitioners chatter about concepts such as 'evidence', 'effectiveness', 'measurement' and 'rigour'. NICE even appoints a professor of clinical pharmacology as its chair – someone who wears a white coat, does ward rounds and used to work in a laboratory. But like the cargo-cult, it is just a facade. It superficially looks like science but it just doesn't work – no cumulative, 'reliable knowledge' results. No planes land.

The reason is that essential elements are missing from the recipe. As explained above, the processes of science and of NICE are profoundly different – one is democratic, the other autocratic; one is oriented toward practice, the other to policy; one is tested against the natural world, the other against political expediency. Feynman suggests that the crucial missing attribute in cargo-cult science is an attitude of integrity and honesty about real world results, and certainly this integrity is lacking in managerial discourse (as Feynman discovered when he investigated the space shuttle *Challenger* disaster (1988)).

In contrast to the ethic of honesty which necessarily permeates scientific practice (Bronowski 1975), NICE already exemplifies a fundamental evasiveness. For instance, by conflating effectiveness with cost-effectiveness in its mission statement, NICE perpetrates the basic dishonesty of implying that these quite distinct variables can be routinely satisfied by a single recommendation. The first NICE decision to disallow the anti-flu drug Relenza (zanamivir) likewise used criteria manufactured *ad hoc* for the purpose of rationalising a politically motivated decision. And what about the acronym NICE? That Orwellian nomenclature speaks volumes about an organisation based upon spin-doctoring rather than patient-doctoring.

The parable of the notebooks

NICE presents itself as a scientific organisation, merely implementing the objectively compelling results of data analysis – hence it claims the objectivity and impartiality of a scientific process. But NICE is almost the opposite of science, because it reverses the relationship between theory and practical experience. Science sees theory as conjectural *explanations* with testable consequences to be measured up against practical experience under controlled conditions. NICE, by contrast, sees theory as *technique* and seeks not to explain, but to excuse – specifically to fabricate excuses for the centralised control of medical practice.

Because it is a matter of applying technique to data in order to support decision, Infostat management creates the impression of being able to *manufacture knowledge* from data. This is reminiscent of the parable told by Karl Popper and quoted by Jacob Bronowski (1975). A man spent his whole life making detailed observations of the world and writing them into notebook after notebook – a meticulous record, leaving out nothing. Humidity levels, racing results, cosmic radiation, the stock market – all were included in his compilation. Many hundreds of these thick notebooks were bequeathed to the Royal Society on his death, for the use of the premier scientists of the nation. But the secretary of the Royal Society read the bequest, took one swift glance at the accumulated volumes, then promptly ordered that the whole lot be dumped into landfill site ...

Why? Well, the moral of the story is that the secretary of the Royal Society knew, without even looking, that the contents of the notebooks must be scientifically worthless. Science is in the questions asked and the means by which they are addressed; it is not an undiscriminating process of relentless, cumulative, impartial observation. Science is not a loose-leaf folder of facts, but the structured knowledge of principles that give rise to the facts – the hidden likeness which explains observations and not the observations themselves. And the application of statistical procedures to such notebooks would not affect the issue – condensed garbage is still garbage.

Infostat management – of which NICE is by far the most extreme example so far – shares the misguided approach of this unfortunate diarist. NICE is a diabolical engine that manufactures decisions when fed with data. These decisions are legitimated – not by the quality of the evidence nor by the patterns revealed by analysis – but by burying the opposition under a heap of misleading information and statistical obfuscation, and by intimidating dissent through the sanctions that will undoubtedly be deployed by CHI. Real medical knowledge does not come to order, nor can it be accelerated by 'fast track' timetables. Its pace is dictated by the natural history of disease and the experience of active practitioners. We know no other valid way and no amount of pretence to the contrary will change that.

Of course, neither I nor anyone else can prove conclusively that good medicine *cannot* be practised using a pseudo-objective system of data-excused management such as NICE. But such a requirement is absurd – it is logically equivalent to asking for proof that the Loch Ness monster *cannot* exist. The present system of medical practice by highly autonomous doctors is already in place, and works to a high level of effectiveness and efficiency, and gives (according to available data) a remarkably high level of public satisfaction. It needs to be improved – but improved by provision of more health *services*, not by cutting and hamstringing services in order to increase managerial control mechanisms. Doctors are far from perfect, but patients would rather trust the judgement of *their* doctors than a government bureaucracy.

The effectiveness and efficiency of health care imposed by diktat from NICE and CHI are purely theoretical, and there is no reason to assume that they will work. The onus of proof lies with those who suggest that an Infostat-fuelled, guideline-generating sausage machine forms a better model for medical practice than that which currently operates.

Conclusions

NICE is not about science, it is about Government and managers attaining the statutory power to control doctors. The aspirations and supposed benefits of NICE do not stand up to a moment's consideration. Its scientific rhetoric is merely an excuse for coercion, its scientific rationale merely the trappings of a 'cargo-cult'. We already know how to do science (Hull 1988), and it is not done like NICE. Top-down regulation based on Infostat technologies is a branch a management theory, not of human biology. Political expediency will corrupt science.

NICE is just part of the NHS sausage machine, a mechanism which exists to support policy decisions and which has little incentive to seek the scientific truth. The policy sausage machine was designed and paid for by politicians, and it will be influenced primarily by politicians. Whatever the phoney feel-good mission statements about 'clinical excellence' and 'health improvement', the fact is that NICE is a Government-funded bureaucracy, and will behave exactly how we expect Government-funded bureaucracies to behave. In other words, NICE will make recommendations the nature of which will be excused by impressive-sounding statistics; but the real point of NICE is not what is in the recommendations, but the fact that there *are* recommendations and the fact that these recommendations will be enforced on doctors by the CHI inquisitors.

Since the real function of NICE and CHI is to control the medical workforce, as long as there *are* recommendations to be enforced by CHI, then NICE will be serving its political purpose. So NICE will control by persuasion, and CHI by intimidation – by carrots and whips. And these are big whips.

T D Lysenko was a Soviet biologist to whom Stalin granted the power to enforce his theories upon fellow biologists (Joravsky 1970). From approximately 1927 to

1964, Lysenko ruled his discipline using the draconian methods of a totalitarian state. Biological science was virtually destroyed, and replaced by data fabrication in the service of propaganda – great agricultural progress was claimed: meanwhile the peasants starved. Disobedient scientists who criticised or resisted were removed from their posts – some were imprisoned and killed.

NICE is not like that – the proposal is only that doctors who disobey NICE recommendations will be harassed, humiliated, sacked or struck off the medical register. CHI will only remove their livelihood, not their lives.

We are assured that NICE and CHI will deploy their powers responsibly, and that sanctions will be used only on those people who really deserve them. The individuals who make such assurances may well be sincere. But once NICE and CHI have power over medical practice, we will be reliant entirely on their sense of restraint to prevent abuses.

Probably, the threat of sanctions will be enough to ensure compliance. Like Galileo, doctors will merely be *shown* the instruments of torture. NICE and CHI can rely on their imaginations to do the rest.

References

Bailar JC 3rd (1997). The promise and problems of meta analysis. *New England Journal of Medicine* **337**, 559–61.

Bronowski J (1975). *Science and human values.* Harper Colophon, New York, USA.

Charlton BG (1993). Management of science. *Lancet* **342**, 99–100.

Charlton BG (1996a). Megatrials are based on a methodological mistake. *British Journal of General Practice* **46**, 429–31.

Charlton BG (1996b). The uses and abuses of meta-analysis. *Family Practice* **13**, 397–401.

Charlton BG (1996). The future of clinical research: from megatrials towards methodological rigour and representative sampling. *Journal of Evaluation in Clinical Practice* **2**, 159–69.

Charlton BG (1997). Restoring the balance: evidence-based medicine put in its place. *Journal of Evaluation in Clinical Practice* **3**, 87–98.

Charlton BG (1999). The ideology of accountability. *Journal of the Royal College of Physicians of London* **33**, 33–5.

Charlton BG & Miles A (1998). The rise and fall of EBM. *QJM* **91**, 371–4.

Feinstein AR (1995). Meta-analysis: statistical alchemy for the 21st century. *Journal of Clinical Epidemiology* **48**, 71–9.

Feynman RP (1986). *'Surely you're joking Mr Feynman'.* Unwin, London.

Feynman RP (1988). *'What do you care what other people think'.* Unwin, London.

Goodman NW (1998). Anaesthesia and evidence-based medicine. *Anaesthesia* **53**, 353–68.

Goodman NW (1999). Who will challenge evidence-based medicine? *Journal of the Royal College of Physicians of London* **33**, 249–51

Griffiths R (1983). *Report of the NHS management inquiry.* DHSS, London.

Hull DL (1988). *Science as a process – an evolutionary account of the social and conceptual development of science.* University of Chicago Press, Chicago (Ill.), USA.

Jenkins S (1995). *Accountable to none – the Tory nationalization of Britain.* Hamish Hamilton, London.

Joravsky D (1970). *The Lysenko affair.* Harvard University Press, Cambridge (MA), USA.

Judson HF (1979). *The eighth day of creation: makers of the revolution in biology.* Jonathan Cape, London.

Julian DG (1995). Secondary prophylaxis after myocardial infarction. *BMJ* **310**, 61.

Klein R (1989). *The politics of the National Health Service* (2nd edition). Longman, London.

Le Fanu J (1999). *The rise and fall of Western medicine.* Little, Brown and Co., London.

Machiavelli N. *The prince* (WK Marriott translator, 1992) David Campbell, London.

Miles A, Bentley P, Polychronis A & Grey J (1997). Evidence-based medicine. Why all the fuss? This is why. *Journal of Evaluation in Clinical Practice* **3**, 83–6.

Miles A, Bentley P, Polychronis A, Grey J & Price N (1998). Recent progress in health services research: on the need for evidence-based debate. *Journal of Evaluation in Clinical Practice* **4**, 257–65.

Miles A, Bentley P, Polychronis A, Grey J & Price N (2000a). Evidence-based healthcare in the new millennium. *Journal of Evaluation in Clinical Practice* **6** (in press).

Miles A, Hill A & Hurwitz B (eds.) (2000b). *Clinical governance: enabling excellence or imposing control?* Aesculapius Medical Press, London (in press).

Oakeshott M (1962). *Rationalism in politics and other essays.* Methuen, London.

Peters T (1989). *Thriving on chaos: handbook for a managerial revolution.* Pan, London.

Sackett DL, Haynes RB & Tugwell P (1985). *Clinical epidemiology.* Little, Brown & Co., Boston (MA), USA.

Ziman J (1978). *Reliable knowledge: an exploration of the ground for belief in science.* Cambridge University Press, Cambridge.

Chapter 3

NICE and the new command structure: with what competence and with what authority will evidence be selected and interpreted for local clinical practice?

Neville W Goodman

Introduction

Change cannot be separated from the reasons for change; nor can those reasons be separated from the circumstances. I started to write this chapter at the end of a week during which the Prime Minister, Mr Blair, criticised public sector workers for stubbornly resisting change. Medicine in Britain is undergoing change for political reasons, which cannot be ignored when considering the recent developments in the structure of medicine. There have been calls to avoid rhetoric (Miles *et al.* 1999) and deal just with facts, logic and evidence. That is not possible in something as complex as health care (Marinker 1994). When a report concluded that breast screening was not worthwhile for women aged below 50, the US Senate voted 96–0 in favour of funding a screening programme (Fletcher 1997). In the big picture of medicine, away from our daily contacts with our patients, politics is impossible to avoid, and is probably the most important factor for how the NHS will develop. This is not to say that politicians themselves will have the largest influence, but that the largest influence will be the result of political discussions between the various interested groups.

A parallel can be drawn with transport. Seven people died when a train belonging to Great Western Railways crashed at Southall in Middlesex. This was not followed by widespread outrage that those seven deaths should have prevented by lessons learned from the earlier ferry disaster involving the *Herald of Free Enterprise*.

What applies to transport does not apply to medicine. Poor medical practice, it seems, is poor medical practice. Children dying after cardiac surgery, general practitioners missing cases of meningitis, and screening laboratories overlooking cases of cancer are linked, implicitly or explicitly, as if it is obvious that they indicate a general rottenness at the heart of the NHS. Faced with this belief, or because it suits politicians to foster this belief, what we are seeing is the political idea that all the difficulties can be solved by something akin to the physicists' grand unifying theory, which currently goes under the name of clinical governance (Goodman 1998b; Miles *et al.* 2000). The irony is that while these various medical failings probably do not share a common theme and therefore a common solution, train and ferry deaths were directly (even if not completely) due to the common theme of profits being put before public safety.

Change, reasons and circumstances

The time of the British Medical Association (BMA) annual conference gives ample opportunity for soundbites, which was when Mr Blair expressed his exasperation that 'the public sector won't change'. This broad-brush statement is impossible to refute, for we were presented with no argument to counter and no evidence to contradict. One of the stimuli to Mr Blair's opinion is the consistent opposition from doctors and other groups in the NHS to the Private Finance Initiative (PFI), a disagreement largely conducted rhetorically. In the week of the 1999 conference, the *BMJ* published an editorial (Smith 1999c) heralding a series of four articles critically analysing the effect of the PFI on the NHS. Saying, as they did, that the initiative was an expensive way of building hospitals, which appeared to cost less only because the true cost was delayed 30 years and included a hidden cost of bed closures, it would not be unfair to describe the conclusions of the authors of the articles as damning. Mr Blair paused long enough only for his speech writers, not long enough for re-analysis. At the time of his response, only the first article had been published. Mr Blair's response was that New Labour would not be swayed by ideology from its purpose of 'modernisation' of the NHS.

This is language on its head: the true mark of the politician. A Conservative health minister once said, 'We need to define the parameters of health care', a statement notable for being truly meaningless (Goodman 1993), unless we know what he meant by parameters. Mr Blair is making the parameters clear: when presented with evidence (to which counter-evidence could be presented, or analysis that the evidence is flawed), he dismisses it as ideology.

Why, then, should anyone be surprised that there are those who describe NICE, CHI and clinical governance as mirages and chimeras? These words are metaphors, with clear meanings: things that appear real but are not; and a mythical beast made up of parts from different animals. The NHS is engaged not in a struggle of conflicting evidence, but in a struggle of conflicting ideologies. Mr Blair accused the BMA of being the doctors' trade union, protecting doctors and ignoring patients (politicians are fond of harking back to the BMA's objections at the founding of the NHS); he suggested that the Government thinks of everyone (Hibbs 1999). Is there any group of humans which does not, in some sense, protect its vested interests? Having asked that rhetorical question, I suggest that politicians have a driving interest in the retention of power, which underlies their every action.

These are the circumstances of the change: a government and civil service (which includes senior public health doctors) giving the impression that they inherently distrust coalface doctors and want to control them. But these circumstances have probably always been so. The reasons for the change are more immediate. They are complex but simply stated, and I have already referred to them: doctors have always made mistakes, but some recent mistakes have been obvious and have been picked up by the media. This has not always been so. Some time in the last 30 years, the media realised the news value of doctors making mistakes. The politicians have turned this to their advantage. The Chief Medical Officer, Professor Liam Donaldson (1999), connecting clinical governance directly to the GMC hearing into children's heart surgery in Bristol, wrote that the affair 'must be seen as a watershed in attitudes towards poor clinical performance'. This quote poses two important questions.

The first question is by whom is it seen as a watershed? It is undoubtedly true that patients due for cardiac surgery in Bristol were worried; it may be true that patients due for cardiac surgery elsewhere in the country were worried; but it is not true that all or even many patients suddenly became more worried about the standard of their medical care. (Another irony is that many disasters are end-results that precipitate instant change. Ferry bookings were cancelled just after the *Herald of Free Enterprise* sank, but this was just the time to go on a ferry because everyone was taking extra care. For children's heart surgery, parents may well still be worried, but once the affair had come to light, Bristol's results in children's heart surgery became among the best in the country. The ironies continue in increased lay involvement in the GMC. The GMC is being pressured to admit more lay members. It is arguable that lay opinion was needed most in the past, when the GMC judged mainly the sexual and commercial mores of doctors.)

A second question posed – or more correctly, begged – is whether poor clinical performance was the true cause of what became the scandal. Other causes were institutional problems driven by political imperatives (Klein 1998), and failure to react to information (Willis 1998). The apportioning of causation may be clearer when the report of the current inquiry is eventually published.

Structures for change

Some structures intended to improve health care, such as the mechanisms for achieving a better balance between consultants and trainee doctors, for reducing the hours of work of trainees, and for continuing medical education (since renamed 'continuing professional development'), have made sense, though have proved difficult to implement. Others, such as clinical audit and evidence-based medicine, make sense at first sight but have serious flaws (Miles *et al.* 1995, 1997, 1998), consistently denied or ignored by some of their enthusiasts. These structures have inevitably brought guidelines into prominence, and now they too have been taken over by structure in NICE. As I write, NICE has done little except reject Relenza (zanamivir) via a 'fast-track' assessment, which has generated substantial controversy, though its chairman has written a great deal about what it will do (Rawlins 1999), and a chief executive and clinical director and communications manager have been appointed. As a coalface clinician, I note that the clinical director is a professor of public health. (Interestingly, the *BMJ* news item reporting the appointment was immediately above another item about a survey of consultant general surgeons. Even before the extra work of clinical governance, 71 per cent of these surgeons are working twice the recommended core hours, and 24 per cent are working up to 60 hours per week.)

The structures, and we could include re-accreditation and revalidation of consultants, do not form a hierarchy, but in clinical governance they are interlinked. Donaldson

(1999) lists six ways in which clinical governance will affect individual practitioners. One is by their 'being aware of best practice guidelines from NICE and other sources and adopting them as part of clinical audit or individual practice developments'. I realise that there is intended to be more to clinical governance than doctors adhering to guidelines, and that NICE intends to help all health professionals and not just doctors. Nonetheless, guidelines to best treatment or to preferred treatment, however it is expressed, are central and likely to have a large effect on how doctors practise medicine in the future.

The lure of evidence-based medicine

All medical treatment should be based on evidence, but I distinguish 'medicine based on evidence' from 'evidence-based medicine' (EBM). By EBM, I mean medicine based on the formal searching for and collecting of data (largely) from randomised controlled trials (RCTs). These trials are seen as the best form of primary evidence, and their subsequent meta-analysis for systematic review underpins preferred treatment. The current fashion is to regard EBM as the safest basis for clinical guidelines.

However, views on the value of EBM are, literally, poles apart: contrast the view that the 'knowledgeable, thoughtful, traditional review remains the closest thing we have to a gold standard of summarizing disparate evidence in medicine' (Bailar 1998, p.62) with the belief that '... [meta-analysis] is clearly superior to the narrative approach to reviewing medical research' (Davey Smith *et al.* 1998, p.224).

I prefer to see EBM as one way of obtaining information about treatments, which under some circumstances is useful. Within my experience, the closer a health service worker is to treating patients, the less enthusiastic they are likely to be about EBM as the only, or at least the best, basis for treatments. One of the worrying aspects of EBM is that it is intuitively appealing. It is not easy to explain the problems of EBM to members of trust boards and other influential non-medical personnel. Surely, they ask, if all the clinical information about a treatment is gathered together in a systematic uniform way, an answer will emerge. This is, of course, true. What is more, the answer can be expressed with clarity and authority. These properties, however, do not confer accuracy or truth.

The journals are replete with articles reporting the conclusions of EBM, and there are books teaching the steps of EBM (Charlton 1997a). There is little written to suggest why EBM, beyond its intuitive appeal, should be reliable, and EBM *has certainly not been tested*. Norman (1999) is not the first to point out the irony that advocates of EBM put their trust in evidence, yet without evidence that EBM works (Miles *et al.* 1997, 1998, 1999). A comparison of meta-analyses and megatrials of the same therapies (LeLorier *et al.* 1997) stimulated heated debate in the journals (see Goodman (1999) for detail), including the comment that later comparison is invalid because the whole point of meta-analysis is to consider the totality of the evidence (Naylor *et al.* 1998). This seems to deny that EBM is testable.

On the other hand, many people have written of the inherent problems of EBM, and their criticisms remain unanswered. The mechanics of EBM are well described, but its philosophical framework is lacking (Hampton 1998).

A really basic problem is that information collected from populations is being applied to individual patients: 'The basic error of EBM is quite simple. It is that epidemiological data do not provide the information necessary to treat individual patients. The error is intractable and intrinsic to the methodological nature of epidemiology, and no amount of statistical jiggery-pokery with huge data sets can make any difference' (Charlton 1997a, p.169[1]). A much-cited paper for the critics of EBM, but not for its advocates, is one in which Feinstein (1994) describes how clinical medicine has been distracted by quantitative models. Kleinert (1998) has the same worry: 'The modern trend to search for precise answers in the form of numbers and probabilities can have only a limited role in human sciences such as medicine'. Feinstein has been cited so many times that one has to ask why there have been, so far as I am aware, no formal refutations of his ideas by those who wish us to practise EBM. In Ghali *et al.*'s (1999) attempt to justify EBM, they do not refute Feinstein, although they do cite some critical references. They do not, however, examine those critics' arguments, but argue by inference that EBM should improve outcome because 'lower' [sic] levels of evidence have been shown to do so. This still fails to answer why *epidemiological* evidence – which may also be of poor or unknown quality – should work for individual patients.

Feinstein himself acknowledges that randomised trials have provided answers in clinical medicine, but mainly about 'therapeutic agents whose *average* efficacy has been unequivocally shown' [emphasis added]. It is the idea of the *average* efficacy that misleads. If the variability around that average is wide, what is the evidence that we do the greatest good for the greatest number by giving everyone the average? This might be so if the differences between patients were random, but they are not. Patients differ systematically from one another (Charlton 1997b). In the present state of clinical knowledge, often we do not know what these systematic differences are. Sometimes, when we choose a treatment for a patient, we employ clinical judgement to make estimates about these differences. Feinstein, who probably has a better understanding of quantitative models than most clinicians, including many who rely on EBM, is a firm advocate of clinical judgement.

Of course, if the variability around the average is not wide, then we can be more confident about preferred treatment – and EBM becomes unnecessary because it takes few patients to know what the average is. The seduction of EBM is that, *statistically,* the bigger the database from which our average is constructed, the more confidence we have in *what the average is*, but this does not make the average applicable to more patients. Marinker (1994, p.5) writes that this mindset leads to 'rational prescribing … expressed as the achievement of mean values, as though there were some evident democratic virtue in the average of irrational behaviours'.

---

1. I have used this quotation elsewhere, in articles that readers should refer to for other similar references (Goodman 1998a, 1999).

What emerges from EBM is only a statistical best estimate. Provided this is sensibly acknowledged, there is nothing inherently wrong with it, but there are other limitations. Much of the work involved in EBM depends on computers. Without them, searching for the evidence would be impossibly laborious and meta-analysis extremely difficult. In computing terms, the input to EBM is data from trials and the output is the computation of meta-analysis. Neither input nor output is necessarily valid.

RCTs – powerful but flawed; meta-analysis – flawed but powerful

RCTs are – in theory – a powerful method of determining which tested treatments have the greatest effect, but they have weaknesses. The conditions of RCTs are not the conditions of clinical practice. For example, much of anaesthesia research is into relief of post-operative pain. Patients who become subjects in these trials get more attention, from clinicians and research nurses, than patients having similar operations but who are not in trials. When we take the results of such trials, however convincing, as a basis for our prescriptions, we cannot prescribe the extra attention. The 'proven' advantage of surgery as treatment for carotid artery stenosis requires to be interpreted in the light of a 9.8 per cent complication rate in community practice, which compares with the 3.7 per cent complication rate in the trials (Swales 1998). The death rate in clinical trials of treatment for myocardial infarction is consistently lower than in hospital practice, despite the introduction of 'proven' treatments (Brown *et al.* 1997).

A common response from those unfamiliar with the conditions under which clinicians work is a sense of indignation that a treatment which *can* be made to work seems unavailable to most patients. This is not just a matter of resources. There are other ways in which randomised trials fail to tell the truth. One is that the constraints on the patients entered into trials are often very tight, which means that the result of the trial may not be applicable to the population from which they were drawn, or at least to the patients seen in the clinic or hospital ward. Another is the difficulty of assessing the quality of trials. I suspect that most trial-naïve people believe that the likelihood of an answer increases with how well trials are carried out. In general, the opposite is true. Important aspects of quality are the methods and success of randomisation and blinding, and failure of these is likely to over-estimate treatment effects, i.e. is more likely to produce an answer. Other aspects of quality are not so easy to judge and are the subject of much discussion. An editorial comment (Ioannidis *et al.* 1998, p.590) on one description of quality rating (Moher *et al.* 1998) was that the findings 'really cast serious doubts on the validity of current clinical research'.

Without being too harsh on the theoretical strengths of randomised trials, it must be recognised that the input to EBM may be less than perfect. The same is true for the output (even if one dismisses the criticism that epidemiological data cannot be applied to individuals). Meta-analysis, it must be remembered, is not a simple single measurement. Meta-analysis is the generic name for various techniques of combining results. Different meta-analysts have their favoured techniques, and argue with one another about which is best (see Goodman (1999)). People are seeking simplistic solutions to inherently complex problems and 'the danger is that through evidence based medicine we will supply them' (Kerridge *et al.* 1998, p.1153).

No evidence for EBM

It cannot be ignored that EBM was put forward as a completely new way of doing medicine, in which the old authority of the experts' customary practices was to be overturned. Although the original triumphalist feel of EBM (Polychronis *et al.* 1996a, 1996b) has waned somewhat, probably more because the realism of working clinicians has tempered it rather than its reasoned critics have weakened it (Couto 1999; Shahar 1999), I remain to be convinced that EBM is not itself another customary practice, following its own political agenda, and generating its own commercial interests.

The lack of a philosophical framework is a continuing source of worry. There is the view within EBM circles that clinical data are the only important basis of clinical practice. This is expressed as an impatience with 'data-free arguments', i.e. there can be no discussion about a treatment's effectiveness or ineffectiveness unless there are data from clinical research. This raises two important points. First, there are large areas of medicine for which clinical data do not exist and are unlikely to exist in the near future (Naylor 1995; Newton *et al.* 1996). This lack of evidence must not be mistaken for lack of effort, or for that area's unworthiness. Kerridge *et al.* (1998) worry that unresearched areas of medicine will be systematically ignored, 'without substantial evidence' becoming 'without substantial value'. Of course, EBM can highlight where evidence is lacking; indeed, some see EBM only as a good way of formulating hypotheses and designing conclusive studies (Blinkhorn 1998). However, although a research agenda is needed before research can start, whether it does start depends on many factors beyond the control of those who wish to do it, or those who wish it done.

The second point has deeper repercussions: 'no data-free arguments' is another intuitively appealing idea, but it is being applied to forms of alternative medicine that have no basis in our modern understanding of anatomy and physiology. A common feature to these forms of practice is explanation of effect by the 'unblocking of energy channels', or other explanations that can only be described as mumbo-jumbo. There are plenty of effective medical treatments for which we have no clear biological explanation; general anaesthesia is one. But, to take general anaesthesia, we may not know how it works, but work it unequivocally does. For that matter, we do not understand gravity, but apples always fall towards the ground. There will always be clinical trials suggestive of an effect of alternative therapies, because that is the nature of probability. Such trials are a constant reminder that randomised clinical trials do not always tell the truth. It is a denial of science to require data and EBM before discounting alternative therapies as effective treatment; it is the antithesis of the scientific basis of medical treatments, and turns back the last 300 years of scientific progress in medicine.

Will guidelines be soundly based?

A political solution is being sought; EBM is attractive to politicians as a basis for practice guidelines, but it is flawed. Is there a more secure way of getting evidence?

This question lacks a universal answer. There is no alternative to looking at appropriate evidence of outcomes for each clinical question. There are general ways of proceeding, but at each stage there are sources of disagreement: what, for example, is *appropriate* evidence? At a meeting convened to discuss the permanent vegetative state, participants were told that any resulting advice offered by the Department of Health would have to be 'evidence-based'. Black (1998, p.25) commented that this might be the ideal, but for conditions such as permanent vegetative state this 'scarcely corresponds to reality, unless one stretches "evidence" to include ... common sense'. At a more definable level than common sense, how does evidence on outcome of benefit balance evidence on outcome of harm and evidence on outcome of cost?

We still do not know exactly how NICE intends to appraise health technologies. Those of us who fear undue subservience to EBM tend to think of EBM whenever we read the words 'evidence-based' or 'systematic', although this may be inference not implication. However, Radford & Rawlins (1999) see NICE as providing a coherent, systematic approach to the appraisal of research evidence. They are critical of 'numerous bodies' issuing guidance in the past who have used different approaches to appraise the evidence. Silverman (1985, p.ix) describes as 'simplistic' the idea that 'there is a fixed set of directions that may be applied mechanically to test a given question'. There are ways – not *a single way* – of balancing outcomes, leaving aside any remaining uncertainty about the benefit, harm and cost, or the measurement of them.

Foremost in any consideration of outcomes research must be the realisation that facts rarely come value-free. It is inevitable that the beliefs and values of the researchers will have an effect, and interpretation depends on point of view (Veatch 1998; Sniderman 1999). One only has to follow the correspondence columns in the journals to realise this (and it is disturbing to remember that critical letters are seldom acknowledged in later citation). Clinical decisions are based on the results of randomised controlled trials and on consensus statements because these processes are seen as detached and objective, but 'no process rises above the people involved'. This is bound to apply to NICE as much as it does to any other consensus. Veatch's conclusion is awkwardly simple: technology assessment is necessarily value-laden.

Clinical science need not feel in any way debased by these disagreements and why they occur; values pervade the whole of science (which is, after all, a human activity) (Collins *et al.* 1994). Experiments (among which we can include clinical trials) are useful only if they are competently done, but when there is controversy, 'no-one can agree on a criterion of competence ... scientists disagree not only about results, but also about the quality of each other's work' (ibid., p.3). There are plenty of examples in science of experimenters regarding the failure of others to replicate the original results as evidence that the replication was faulty; this same failure is taken by the replicators as evidence that the original observations were faulty. Experiments alone are not capable of settling all issues. In extreme cases, this leads to public arguments between scientists, the sides expressing mutually exclusive certainty. Many people are uneasy that science is uncertain, but for science to question things it is almost a requirement that it be uncertain. People are even more uneasy that clinical science is uncertain, and that values may affect it, but they must learn to live with uncertainty.

Outcomes, presentation and consensus

Even if outcome data are robust, they are only part of the patient-doctor consultation (Willems 1998); for much of what doctors do, there are no reliable data on outcomes, and indeed it may be difficult even to define what the outcomes are. Murphy DJ (1998) cites Feinstein (1994) and worries about the measurements we make for outcomes research. He is especially wary of how measurements are reported. He asks which of the following statements is more likely to encourage women to go for breast cancer screening: 'Yearly mammograms reduce the risk of dying by 33 per cent'; or, '7,000 people need to have yearly screenings to avoid one premature cancer death'. Both statements are (within their statistical confidence limits) 'outcome facts'. More recent work (cited by Dickersin (1999)) has been reported under media headlines of mammography for women under 50 'saving lives', and this is true. Of 10,000 40–49-year-olds screened, 30 will be diagnosed with breast cancer and treated. Some of these women would otherwise have died. But these 30 will be from 640 who had abnormal mammograms, of whom 150 had biopsies. Will the women eventually pronounced clear be reassured? Will they be grateful for the worry they went through? How do we measure these factors for outcomes research? Dickersin also points out that some of the 30 women will be treated for an *in-situ* lesion, the natural history of which is unknown.

Fahey *et al.* (1995) presented outcome data to members of UK health authorities, and asked them to choose between four health programmes. Only four of the 140 respondents realised that the four 'programmes' were the same data presented in four different ways. Doctors are misled in the same way, and patients – who have even less understanding than doctors – are misled even more.

Even when the data are gathered and presented, another variable is the process of consensus. There is unease with some of the Department of Health's earlier consensus solutions in health technology. Freemantle & Mason (1999) think the methods used by the regionally funded development and evaluation committees (DEC) are inappropriate. They use some specific examples, and are interested especially in estimating costs per quality-adjusted life year (QALY), but conclude that audit to ensure that the right patient gets the right treatment at the right time is unrealistic, and that simple performance measures are likely to be misleading. There are many (Correspondence 1999a) who disagree fundamentally with them – but that is my point.

Do we need NICE guidelines?

There have been guidelines as long as there has been medicine. Books, reviews and editorials provide guidelines. We need guidelines; allowing for the limitations of the evidence upon which they are based, they are immensely useful. What is altering is the way guidelines are regarded. They have always been, and must remain, a *basis* for action. They are tending to become *prescriptions* for action, but this should be avoided except under certain clearly defined circumstances. Even less must they become rigid measuring devices for assessing the performance of clinicians and other health professionals. Whether they are called guidelines, practice parameters, clinical algorithms, or whatever, guidelines are 'recommendations that can be accepted, rejected, or modified to fit the circumstances of the case at issue' (Shomaker 1995, p.390). Shomaker distinguishes guidelines from standards, defined as minimum requirements to ensure clinically competent care and which carry an implication of compulsion. Vickers (1996), using another term and writing about the practice of anaesthesia, thinks protocols are useful for rare events when action must be quick and correct, and for unfamiliar procedures performed outside normal working that might cause harm; but protocols are themselves harmful for things within normal practice, and for which there is accepted professional discretion. This begs the question what is 'accepted'. It brings us back to the consideration of the evidence upon which practice is based, and to the new Institute's intentions: will NICE be producing guidelines, or standards?

Rawlins (1999, p.1079) wrote that the Institute's output would not be mandatory, which suggests he was writing of guidelines, but that 'health professionals would be wise to record their reasons for non-compliance in patients' medical records', which strongly suggests standards. Radford & Rawlins' (1999) diagram has NICE producing 'standards' of clear service, with CHI (among others) monitoring those standards.

NICE fully realises its inherent difficulties. Rawlins (1999) listed four problems of guidelines, the last of which – that most guidelines are not readily available – is easy to solve for a well-funded central body. The other problems are not so easy to solve and I cannot see how NICE is any more likely to solve them than anyone else. Rawlins (ibid., p.1080) writes that available guidelines are of variable quality, and that 'although some are based on a close and exhaustive review of scientific published work, others are derived from opinion or anecdote'. Implicit in this is that opinion and anecdote are wrong, very much the hard-line EBM stance, and suggesting that meta-analysis will be the exemplar. The difficulties with this have been outlined above and have already been recognised in a previous Government-sponsored report (Murphy MK *et al.* 1998, p.1): 'In an ideal world, clinical guidelines would be based on [rigorous] evidence [but] there are few areas of health care where sufficient research-based evidence exists or may ever exist ... [Guidelines] will inevitably have to be based partly or largely on the opinions and experience of clinicians and others with knowledge'. This report fully acknowledges that even the data may be faulty, and describes the development of consensus as 'mak[ing] the best use of available information', recognising that it is 'inevitably vulnerable to the possibility of capturing collective ignorance' (ibid., p.1).

Another problem Rawlins recognises is that many clinical guidelines covering the same area are contradictory and give divergent advice. Given the nature of medical knowledge, this is inevitable. What will make NICE's guidelines, *ipso facto*, 'better' or more 'correct' than those of a Royal College? De Wildt *et al.* (1999) worry about the 'wave of initiatives' intended to improve professional performance emanating from organisations such as Royal Colleges, primary care groups, NICE, CHI, defence organisations, and the General Medical Council, to which we could add national service frameworks (Anonymous 1999a). It is not yet clear whether NICE will in some way vet or rubber-stamp guidelines originating elsewhere. If its guidelines differ from another organisation's, from whose guidelines should doctors 'record their reasons for non-compliance'? Murphy MK *et al.* (1998, p.2) cite Fletcher in writing that consensus 'rarely resolves disputes where strong disagreement exists'. Under these circumstances, NICE can choose between opinions, but the disputes will remain (during the development of some recent guidelines for treating hypertension, the chairman resigned, though he later rejoined (Anonymous 1999c)): there are only a certain number of experts who can be called on to serve and there will be participants common to other bodies and to the Institute.

Four possible topics for NICE appraisal

I give four examples of the difficulties in bringing evidence together for coherent guidelines. The first is for the management of anticoagulation in atrial fibrillation. After Rosenberg & Donald (cited in Goodman (1998a)) used this therapeutic conundrum as an exercise in EBM and set a target international normalised ratio of 1.5–2.0, they were accused of picking a ratio 'out of thin air', with too narrow a range, and contrary to the then-current guidelines. They countered the criticism by writing, 'We *believe* the lower range to be safer for the patient [added emphasis]' (ibid., p.358) and added (without further evidence) that their local anticoagulation laboratory recommended the narrow range. A few months later, another group set the target ratio at 3.0 because no treatment effect was apparent with anticoagulation below a ratio of 2.0. There are still disagreements (Correspondence 1999c).

A second example is the management of sleep apnoea. There has been a disagreement between clinicians and public health physicians about the treatment of this condition (see Goodman (1998a); Charlton (1999)). The clinicians wrote: 'It would be unfortunate if this review led to patients being denied a cheap and effective treatment [preventing them from] running an increased risk of premature death' (Goodman 1998a, p.361). The public health physicians wanted patients to be 'reassured that assertions about associations [with] disability and death are unfounded or premature' (ibid.). This argument is now probably settled in the clinicians' favour

(Jenkinson *et al.* 1999), although uncertainty about how 'sleep apnoea' is defined should ensure the debate continues (Wright *et al.* 1999).

These two examples pose the same question: what if NICE had reached its conclusion before the later evidence? Can it keep all its guidelines continuously under review? How frequently will clinicians have to check whether the guidelines have changed, and will adherence to an earlier set put the clinicians at risk?

A third example is laparoscopic hernia repair, tested in a recent large multi-centre trial and the subject of a news story in a medical journal (Bower 1999). After laparoscopic repair there was less pain and a quicker return to normal life than after open repair, but the few serious complications and recurrences that occurred did so only after laparoscopy. The leader of the trial concluded that laparoscopic hernia repair is an operation only for specialists. An author of the guidelines on hernia repair produced by the Royal College of Surgeons, not involved in the trial, concluded instead that laparoscopy is a waste of resources, and that repairing hernias does not need specialist surgeons. He believes it is better to use laparoscopy for operations where the technique makes a real difference. How could NICE decide between these views?

The fourth example featured in the media announcements when NICE started work in August 1999. One of its first tasks was to appraise interferon for multiple sclerosis. An article in *Drugs and Therapeutics Bulletin* (Anonymous 1996) suggested interferon should not be given unless in a trial or under strict audit. In the same year, the NHS Executive was criticised in an editorial (Richards 1996) for accepting interferon treatment, contradicting that article and the opinion of the Association of British Neurologists. The editorial provoked dissenting views (Correspondence 1997), some from pressure groups, others questioning the studies on which the conclusions were based. McKee (1998) wrote that interferon produced only small benefits, and Ferner (1996) suggested it would be better to spend the estimated £10,000 per patient per year on better services for patients with multiple sclerosis. This was the conclusion also of an NHS Health Technology Assessment (HTA) report (Parkin *et al.* 1998), so a Government-sponsored body has already appraised the evidence. Another *Drugs and Therapeutics Bulletin* (Anonymous 1998) criticised a manufacturer's claim of effect, and did not change the earlier conclusion that routine use was not appropriate. Goodkin (1998), writing from a centre for multiple sclerosis in the USA, thought interferon should be available immediately for certain patients. Among letters in the *Lancet* (Correspondence 1998) was one coming back to the issue of resources, calculating the cost of interferon for preventing progression as £550,000 per QALY. Surely all this and much more will be familiar to neurologists with an interest in multiple sclerosis, and is part of the evidence that Giovannoni & Miller (1999) used in concluding that 'IFN-β is currently the treatment of choice for patients with relapsing-remitting MS.' Since then Forbes *et al.* (1999) have re-inforced the view that money would be better spent improving patients' quality of life in other ways.

What decision is NICE to make that will help neurologists? (I will not consider here the action to take about neurologists unfamiliar with the evidence but treating multiple sclerosis.) Unless additional clinical evidence becomes available – and perhaps even if it does – the decision on interferon appears to me, as an impartial observer, to be, not medical, but societal and involving value judgements. NICE (or anyone else, or any other body) has no monopoly on value judgements. Michael Gross, among further correspondence on the subject (Correspondence 1999b), hopes that NICE will look not just at the scientific evidence and price, but at the moral, ethical and legal issues. Gross asks too much: no national body can make decisions on moral and ethical issues of medical treatment that can apply to an individual patient treated according to evidence-based (however evidence be interpreted) guidelines from which clinicians would be 'wise to record … non-compliance', and Rawlins (1999) gave no indication that NICE would base decisions on those grounds.

Rawlins did see NICE making decisions on cost-effectiveness and stopping 'postcode prescribing', which sits oddly with his denial that NICE would be involved in rationing health care. Either a treatment is effective, or it is not. If a treatment is effective but expensive, then an equally effective but less expensive treatment should be used. The reason for postcode prescribing is that some treatments are expensive but without alternative, and in different parts of the country different expensive diseases are favoured. We clearly cannot (or will not) afford all these expensive treatments for expensive diseases, so my interpretation is that rationing (or choosing priorities) will be by disease instead of by geographical area.

I agree with Horton's (1999) editorial comment that NICE is trying to do too much, and that it is skirting the issue of rationing. Horton also noted that the 30–50 technologies to be assessed each year will be picked by the Department of Health, which risks choice of disease and treatment by 'focus groups of floating voters in marginal constituencies or treasury accountants'. He also asked – while being generally optimistic about NICE – a series of other questions, including what the criteria of cost-effectiveness will be, and how the pharmaceutical industry will be kept at arm's length.

In another editorial comment, Smith (1999b) made the same point as Horton that NICE cannot possibly do what it intends, and asked how new treatments can be evaluated without considering treatments already in use. Smith quoted from an interview with Rawlins in the *BMA News Review* (Coulson 1999) in which Rawlins foresaw doctors going to work with the British National Formulary in one pocket and NICE guidelines in the other; Smith commented wryly that a wheelbarrow would be more realistic.

I find it disturbing that, in common with the lack of response from advocates of EBM, these editorial comments demanded a response but did not seem to get one. Rawlins, with Radford, who is head of the NHSE Public Health Development Unit, wrote a later article about NICE (Radford *et al.* 1999). This article cited only Department of Health publications, failing completely to mention the specific problems raised by Smith and Horton, and it is unlikely theirs were the only critical comments. It is as if repeating all the good things that NICE intends will in some way make them happen. I, for one, would be interested to hear on what evidence Rawlins (1999, p.1082) based his statement that NICE 'will decrease ... costs ... [for] ischaemic heart disease'.

Conclusion

There is nothing wrong with NICE, except that its declared primary purpose makes it simply unnecessary. Whatever one thinks of EBM, it has brought the idea of the proper assessment of evidence well to the fore, and we have plenty of groups producing guidelines based on evidence of one sort or another. On page 336 of the same issue of the *Journal of the Royal College of Physicians* as the articles on multiple sclerosis (Giovannoni *et al.* 1999) and NICE (Radford *et al.* 1999) was an advertisement for a 50-page report of a working party of the Royal College of Physicians, titled *Domiciliary oxygen therapy services. Clinical guidelines and advice for prescribers.* We do not need NICE to tell us how to give domiciliary oxygen; the physicians have done that. Nor does NICE need to appraise the use of interferon for multiple sclerosis, the HTA has done that (see above). Rawlins writes that the products of the NHS HTA programme will be an important starting point for the Institute's activities, but NICE seems to be starting by starting all over again. What we need is someone to tell us whether to prescribe domiciliary oxygen for chronic pulmonary disease or, instead, prescribe interferon for multiple sclerosis. Rawlins mentions concerns with priorities in the last paragraph of his article, almost as a throwaway, but to me it should be the most important function of NICE. When the acronym stands for the National Institute for Clinical *Excellence*, this is difficult. If a disease or treatment fails to become a priority, the affected patients will not have experienced excellence however excellently patients with other conditions have been treated. In a Department of Health circular (1999), a Freudian slip transformed NICE to National Institute for Clinical *Effectiveness* (which is what many clinicians think NICE stands for, anyway); this is a better term but, as I have argued, not what we need. What we do need is an explicit National Institute for Clinical Expediency, using expediency in the sense of good policy, pragmatism and utilitarianism rather than opportunism and self-seeking.

Even if NICE does what it intends, even if I am wrong about the problems of interpreting evidence, even if consensus is less difficult than we believe, the battle will still be lost. All the structures being applied to the NHS are perceived as the answer to poor medical practice (among other deficiencies). It does not matter whether this perception is true or not, because the media are not interested in 'fairness, balance or even the veracity of the reporting' (Davies *et al.* 1999); they are only interested in bad practice, and that they will always find. Willis (1999) gives direct personal evidence that the newspapers were not interested in balance in their reporting of the Bristol cardiac affair, and even cites a suggestion that politicians are using the media to damage public respect for doctors. Rayner (1999, p.31) asked:

'Who do these news editors think is going to look after them when they get ill? If the NHS has been fatally flawed by their ill treatment of it, there won't be anyone'.

NICE will improve some medical care in the short term, but it won't save the NHS. In the words of an editorial (Anonymous 1999b, p.4), 'New Labour, it seems, has still to learn that the world is not technically perfectible: that, despite everyone's best efforts, benefit claimants will sometimes cheat, children skive off lessons ... and criminals walk free.' To this could be added, 'and doctors not use the best treatments'. The editorial continued, 'It would be a better government if it sometimes admitted that nothing (or not very much) can or should be done' (ibid., p.4), but it needs the media and the public to let the Government admit it. The only way to avoid the health care ratchet turning is for people to realise that 'death is inevitable; most major diseases cannot be cured; antibiotics are no use for flu; artificial hips wear out; hospitals are dangerous places; drugs all have side effects; most medical treatments achieve only marginal benefits and many don't work at all; screening tests produce false negative results; and there are better ways of spending money than on healthcare technology' (Smith 1999a, p.210).

There are no simple solutions to the problems of health care. While the public disquiet (as opposed to the disquiet of the public) focuses on choices of health technology as the key to future success, it is worth noting that when doctors themselves suffer poor treatment (McCormick 1996), they are rarely critical of technical failure, but of failures of communication, understanding and empathy, failures insoluble by evidence-based guidelines. The Institute's members may be dedicated and determined, but NICE is part of an intuitively simple political answer to an immensely complex set of real problems, which offers the benefit of yet again shifting the responsibility away from the politicians.

References

Anonymous (1996). Interferon beta-1b – hope or hype? *Drugs and Therapeutics Bulletin* **34**, 9–11.

Anonymous (1998). Interferon beta-1A for multiple sclerosis. *Drugs and Therapeutics Bulletin* **36**, 7–8.

Anonymous (1999a). Developing and delivering national service frameworks. *CMO's update* (23), 2.

Anonymous (1999b). Why justice should be inefficient. *New Statesman* 24 May, p.4.

Anonymous (1999c). A pressure to agree. *Lancet* **354**, 787.

Bailar JC 3rd (1998). Meta-analysis and large randomized, controlled trials [Correspondence]. *New England Journal of Medicine* **338**, 62.

Black D (1998). The limitations of evidence. *Journal of the Royal College of Physicians of London* **32**, 23–36.

Blinkhorn S (1998). Is meta better? *Nature* **392**, 671–2.

Bower H (1999). Laparoscopic hernia surgery linked to increased complications. *BMJ* **319**, 211.

Brown N, Young T, Gray D, Skene AM & Hampton JR (1997). Inpatient deaths from acute myocardial infarction 1982–1992: analysis of data in the Nottingham heart attack register. *BMJ* **315**, 159–64.

Charlton BG (1997a). Book review of evidence-based medicine. *Journal of Evaluation in Clinical Practice* **3**, 169–72.

Charlton BG (1997b). Restoring the balance: evidence-based medicine put in its place. *Journal of Evaluation in Clinical Practice* **3**, 87–98.

Charlton BG (1999). Clinical research methods for the new millennium. *Journal of Evaluation in Clinical Practice* **5**, 251–63.

Collins H & Pinch T (1994). *The Golem: what everyone should know about science.* Canto, Cambridge University Press, Cambridge.

Coulson J (1999). NICE work [Interview with Sir Michael Rawlins]. *BMA News Review* 13 Mar, 20–3.

Correspondence (1997). Interferon in multiple sclerosis. *BMJ* **314**, 600–2.

Correspondence (1998). Interferon β therapy for multiple sclerosis. *Lancet* **353**, 494–8.

Correspondence (1999a). Electronic responses to: Not playing with a full DEC: why development and evaluation committee methods for appraising new drugs may be inadequate. Available at: http://www.bmj.com/cgi/eletters/318/7196/1480.

Correspondence (1999b). Interferon beta in multiple sclerosis. *Lancet* **354**, 512–13.

Correspondence (1999c). Managing atrial fibrillation in elderly people. *BMJ* **319**, 452–4.

Couto J S (1999). Evidence-based medicine: a Kuhnian perspective of a transvestite non-theory. *Journal of Evaluation in Clinical Practice* **4**, 267–75.

Davey Smith G & Egger M (1998). Unresolved issues and future developments. *BMJ* **316**, 221–5.

Davies HTO & Shields AV (1999). Public trust and accountability for clinical performance: lessons from the national press reportage of the Bristol hearing. *Journal of Evaluation in Clinical Practice* **5**, 335–42.

de Wildt G, Heath I & Gill P (1999). Performance of doctors. *Lancet* **354**, 165.

Department of Health (1999). *Continuing professional development: quality in the new NHS.* Health Service Circular HSC 1999/54.

Dickersin K (1999). Breast screening in women aged 40–49 years: what next? *Lancet* **353**, 1896–7.

Donaldson L (1999). Clinical governance – medical practice in a new era. *Journal of the Medical Defence Union* **15**, 7–9.

Fahey T, Griffiths S & Peters TJ (1995). Evidence based purchasing: understanding results of clinical trials and systematic reviews. *BMJ* **311**, 1056–60.

Feinstein AR (1994). Clinical judgement revisited: the distraction of quantitative models. *Annals of Internal Medicine* **120**, 799–805.

Ferner RE (1996). Newly licensed drugs. *BMJ* **313**, 1157–8.

Fletcher SW (1997). Whither scientific deliberation in health policy recommendations? *New England Journal of Medicine* **336**, 1180–3.

Forbes RB, Lees A, Waugh N & Swingler RJ (1999). Population-based cost utility study of interferon beta-1b in secondary progressive multiple sclerosis. *BMJ* **319**, 1529–33.

Freemantle N & Mason J (1999). Not playing with a full DEC: why development and evaluation committee methods for appraising new drugs may be inadequate. *BMJ* **318**, 1480–2.

Ghali WA, Saitz R, Sargious PM & Hershman WY (1999). Evidence-based medicine and the real world: understanding the controversy. *Journal of Evaluation of Clinical Practice* **5**, 133–8.

Giovannoni G & Miller DH (1999). Multiple sclerosis and its treatment. *Journal of the Royal College of Physicians of London* **33**, 315–22.

Goodkin DE (1998). Interferon β therapy for multiple sclerosis. *Lancet* **352**, 1486–7.

Goodman NW (1993). Paradigm, parameter, paralysis of mind. *BMJ* **307**, 1627–9.

Goodman NW (1998a). Anaesthesia and evidence-based medicine. *Anaesthesia* **53**, 353–68.

Goodman NW (1998b). Clinical governance. *BMJ* **317**, 1725–7.

Goodman NW (1999). Who will challenge evidence-based medicine? *Journal of the Royal College of Physicians of London* **33**, 249–51.

Hampton JR (1998). Evidence based cardiology. *BMJ* **317**, 1326.

Hibbs J (1999). Blair tells BMA critics that reforms will go on. *Daily Telegraph* 7 July, p.6.

Horton R (1999). NICE: a step forward in the quality of NHS care. *Lancet* **353**, 1028–9.

Ioannidis JPA & Lau J (1998). Can quality of clinical trials and meta-analyses be quantified? *Lancet* **352**, 590–1.

Jenkinson C, Davies RJO, Mullins R & Stradling JR (1999). Comparison of therapeutic and subtherapeutic continuous positive airway pressure for obstructive sleep apnoea: a randomised prospective clinical trial. *Lancet* **353**, 2100–5.

Kerridge I, Lowe M & Henry D (1998). Ethics and evidence based medicine. *BMJ* **316**, 1151–3.

Klein R (1998). Competence, professional self regulation, and the public interest. *BMJ* **316**, 1740–2.

Kleinert S (1998). Rationing of health care – how should it be done? *Lancet* **352**, 1244.

LeLorier J, Grégoire G, Benhaddad A, Lapierre J & Derderian F (1997). Discrepancies between meta-analyses and subsequent large randomized, controlled trials. *New England Journal of Medicine* **337**, 536–42.

Marinker M (1994). Evidence, paradox, and consensus. In *Controversies in health care politics: challenges to practice* (ed. M Marinker), pp.1–24. BMJ Publishing Group, London.

McCormick J (1996). Death of the personal doctor. *Lancet* **348**, 667–8.

McKee L (1998). Interferon beta produces only small benefits in multiple sclerosis. *BMJ* **316**, 1410.

Miles A, Bentley P, Polychronis A, Price N & Grey J (1995). Clinical audit in the National Health Service: fact or fiction? *Journal of Evaluation in Clinical Practice* **2**, 29–35.

Miles A, Bentley P, Polychronis A & Grey J (1997). Evidence-based medicine. Why all the fuss? This is why. *Journal of Evaluation in Clinical Practice* **3**, 83–6.

Miles A, Bentley P, Polychronis A, Grey J & Price N (1998). Recent progress in health services research: on the need for evidence-based debate. *Journal of Evaluation in Clinical Practice* **4**, 257–65.

Miles A, Bentley P, Polychronis A, Grey J & Price N (1999). Advancing the evidence-based healthcare debate. *Journal of Evaluation in Clinical Practice* **5**, 97–101.

Miles A, Hill A & Hurwitz B (eds.) (2000). *Clinical governance: enabling excellence or imposing control?* Aesculapius Medical Press, London (in press).

Moher D, Pham B, Jones A, Cook DJ, Jadad AR, Moher M *et al.* (1998). Does quality of reports of randomised trials affect estimates of intervention efficacy reported in meta-analyses? *Lancet* **352**, 609–13.

Murphy DJ (1998). Guideline glitches: measurements, money, and malpractice. In *Getting doctors to listen: ethics and outcomes data in context* (ed. PJ Boyle), pp.100–10. Georgetown University Press, Washington (DC), USA.

Murphy MK, Black NA, Lamping DL, McKee CM, Sanderson CFB, Askham J *et al.* (1998). Consensus development guidelines, and their use in clinical guideline development. *Health Technology Assessment* **2**(3).

Naylor CD (1995). Grey zones of clinical practice: some limits to evidence-based medicine. *Lancet* **345**, 840–2.

Naylor CD & Davey Smith G (1998). Test meta-analyses for stability. *BMJ* **317**, 206–7.

Newton J & West E (1996). Evidence-based medicine and compassion. *Lancet* **347**, 1839.

Norman GR (1999). Examining the assumptions of evidence-based medicine. *Journal of Evaluation in Clinical Practice* **5**, 139–47.

Parkin D, McNamee P, Jacoby A, Miller P, Thomas S & Bates D (1998). A cost-utility analysis of interferon beta for multiple sclerosis. *Health Technology Assessment* **2**(4).

Polychronis A, Miles A & Bentley P (1996a). Evidence-based medicine: Reference? Dogma? Neologism? New orthodoxy? *Journal of Evaluation in Clinical Practice* **2**, 1–3.

Polychronis A, Miles A & Bentley P (1996b). The protagonists of evidence-based medicine: arrogant, seductive and controversial. *Journal of Evaluation in Clinical Practice* **2**, 9–12.

Radford G & Rawlins M (1999). The National Institute for Clinical Excellence: the government's agenda and the College's role. *Journal of the Royal College of Physicians of London* **33**, 303–4.

Rawlins M (1999). In pursuit of quality: the National Institute for Clinical Excellence. *Lancet* **353**, 1079–82.

Rayner C (1999). How the good news hit the spike. *New Statesman* 26 July, p.31.

Richards RG (1996). Interferon trials in multiple sclerosis. *BMJ* **313**, 1159.

Shahar E (1999). Evidence-based medicine: a new paradigm or the Emperor's new clothes? *Journal of Evaluation in Clinical Practice* **4**, 277–82.

Shomaker TS (1995). Practice policies in anesthesia: a foretaste of practice in the 21st century. *Anesthesia and Analgesia* **80**, 388–403.

Silverman WA (1985). *Human experimentation: a guided step into the unknown.* Oxford University Press, Oxford.

Smith R (1999a). The NHS: possibilities for the endgame. *BMJ* **318**, 209–10.

Smith R (1999b). NICE: a panacea for the NHS? *BMJ* **318**, 823–4.

Smith R (1999c). PFI: perfidious financial idiocy. *BMJ* **319**, 2–3.

Sniderman AD (1999). Clinical trials, consensus conferences, and clinical practice. *Lancet* **354**, 327–30.

Swales J (1998). The National Health Service and the science of evaluation: two anniversaries. *Health Trends* **30**, 20–2.

Veatch RM (1998). Technology assessment: inevitably a value judgement. In *Getting doctors to listen: ethics and outcomes data in context* (ed. PJ Boyle), pp.180–95. Georgetown University Press, Washington (DC), USA.

Vickers M D (1996). Guidelines and protocols. *Today's Anaesthetist* **11**, 84–5.

Willems D (1998). Outcomes, guidelines, and implementation in France, the Netherlands, and Great Britain. In *Getting doctors to listen: ethics and outcomes data in context* (ed. PJ Boyle), pp.153–63. Georgetown University Press, Washington (DC), USA.

Willis JAR (1998). The aftermath of the Bristol case. Case arose through a failure of action, not of detection [Letter]. *BMJ* **317**, 811.

Willis JAR (1999). The pen is mightier than the scalpel. Commentary on the paper – Public trust and accountability for clinical performance: lessons from the national press reportage of the Bristol hearing (HTO Davies & AV Shields, *Journal of Evaluation in Clinical Practice* **5**, 335–42). *Journal of Evaluation in Clinical Practice* **5**, 343–6.

Wright J, Sheldon TA & Watt I (1999). Sleep apnoea. *Lancet* **354**, 600.

Chapter 4

Clinical guidelines for primary care: principles and problems

Gene Feder

Introduction

The contested validity of guidelines, uncertainty about their application to clinical practice and scepticism about their use in national standard-setting are all apparent in many of the contributions to this book. The stances that individual authors take in relation to these issues are in part influenced by their academic disciplines and whether or not they have been implicated in guideline development and implementation, as well as by broader concerns about the direction of health care in the UK. Therefore it is appropriate for me to declare my own background and involvement with guidelines, as well as potential conflicts of interest.

As a general practitioner in east London I am a recipient and periodic user of clinical guidelines. At a local and national level I have been involved in the development of clinical guidelines, moving from documents based on informal consensus to more structured guidelines based on systematic reviews and appraisal of trial evidence. My academic work has included trials of clinical guidelines implementation in primary care (Feder *et al.* 1995) and the validation of a tool for the appraisal of guidelines quality (Littlejohn *et al.* 1999). I have also helped formulate guideline policy, particularly through The Royal College of General Practitioners and through advice to various NHSE committees, the World Health Organization and the pharmaceutical industry. I am an 'insider' with a vested interest in a central role for guidelines in clinical practice. It is from this vantage point that I will discuss the role of guidelines in primary care.

Background

'Pound together: dried wine dregs, juniper and prunes; pour beer on the mixture. Then rub the diseased part with oil and bind on ...' (quoted in Majno 1975, p.46)

Clinical guidelines are not new, as can be seen in the above quote from a Sumerian clay tablet dating from 2100 BC. Explicit guidance (or instructions) from one clinician to another on diagnosis and treatment is intrinsic to the practice of medicine. Yet there are several features of guidance in the form of clinical guidelines that are relatively new and have spread beyond their origins in North American and British medicine:

the scientific validity of guidance, the interest of extra-professional agencies and the implementation of guidance.

There is concern about the scientific validity of guideline recommendations, i.e. the extent to which they are reliably based on research evidence of effective practice. The quest for more valid guidelines is part of a wider move towards basing treatment decisions on clinical trial evidence and the rhetoric of 'evidence-based' practice. Bibliographic databases of published research have revolutionised access to research; systematic review methods have led to less biased summaries of trial results; and guidelines are widely seen as tools for conveying to clinicians recommendations based on these summaries.

Attention to the *implementation* of guidance for effective practice is also relatively recent. It grows directly out of a recognition that even when clinicians are aware of research evidence relevant to their management of patients, often they do not apply it to individual patient care. A long-standing concern with the avoidance of medical negligence is now extended to attempts to update and improve the current practice of most clinicians.

An important concomitant of guideline development was the recognition of variation in the nature and quality of health care for the same conditions within the same health care systems. This, combined with the economic crisis in western health care over the past 25 years, is temporally and causally linked to the development of explicit clinical guidelines. The forces leading to the proliferation of guidelines were not, nor are they today, largely internal to the medical profession. The growing sophistication of patient groups and associations, with improved access to research evidence and ability to challenge clinical policy decisions, has also influenced the development of clinical guidelines, with the inclusion of patient versions. Finally, the pharmaceutical industry has been active in funding the development and production of guidelines as part of a commercial interest in the promotion of their products.

I will return to some of these issues in the context of primary care guidelines.

Principles of primary care guidelines

A widely cited definition of clinical guidelines comes from the Institute of Medicine in the USA (Fields & Lohr 1992, p.14):

> *'Systematically developed statements to assist practitioner and patient decisions about appropriate health care for specific clinical circumstances.'*

The idealistic (in terms of current medical practice) depiction of shared decision-making between clinician and patient makes it more a *desiratum* than a description of how guidelines on either side of the Atlantic are currently used. The individualistic tone of the definition reflects a political function: distancing guidelines from their potential or actual role as a means of defining and controlling the activity of clinicians. It is ironic that US doctors have more experience than British clinicians of the external restriction of practice through clinical guidelines (managed care guidelines from third-party payers).

A recent international definition of guidelines (Woolf *et al.* 1999, p.527) is less challenging, but more grounded in reality:

> *'Official statements from health organisations and agencies on how best to care for medical conditions or to perform clinical procedures.'*

Whereas the US definition places the locus of decision-making between doctor and patient, the latter avoids locating it at all. It also does not attempt to exclude guidance that is developed in a non-systematic way.

There is a growing consensus about the desirable qualities of clinical guidelines, which are now partly reflected in a validated appraisal tool (Cluzeau *et al.* 1999). For the purposes of this chapter, I want to draw attention to four *a priori* principles of effective primary care guidelines: they are based on comprehensive review of relevant research evidence; recommendations are explicitly linked to the evidence; the guidelines are disseminated to primary care teams and implemented in day-to-day practice/clinical decision-making.

There are a number of features of UK primary care that make its clinicians potentially welcome clinical guidelines. First, the wide range of clinical areas for which we are responsible means it is impossible to 'keep up' with the evidence we need in order to make appropriate decisions. Our patients range from neonates to nursing home residents, and the conditions range from acute infections to chronic mental illness. New evidence for effective treatment in any particular clinical area is likely to pass us by or only come to our attention through pharmaceutical industry promotion. Second, the shift of chronic disease management from hospital care to primary care means that complex diagnostic and treatment decisions for patients with, for example, diabetes or coronary heart disease are made by general practitioners. Third, patients are becoming more knowledgeable about their conditions and some are challenging us to work with them as partners in clinical decision-making. It is not unusual today for my consultations to include printouts from websites. Guidelines are potentially useful in engaging patients with high-quality evidence about what is effective and for whom. Fourth, the requirements of clinical governance in primary care entail explicit guidance about quality of care that can be represented in guidelines. These features favour a useful role for clinical guidelines in primary care.

There are other aspects of general practice that make it a less comfortable setting for the application of guidelines (Sweeney 1996). Many of our patients do not fall into discrete diagnostic groups or, indeed, cannot be given a diagnosis at all. Others have multiple conditions that cannot be accommodated in one guideline. Finally, the general practitioner's task goes beyond the bringing of best evidence to the patient's problems and encompasses recognition of the 'uniqueness of the patient's human condition and the significance and gravity of the illness from the patient's perspective' (ibid., p.78). I will return to the implications of this wider task at the end of the chapter, after discussing the nature and use of guidelines to date within primary care, focusing on the problems that we face in their development, dissemination and implementation. These problems need to be addressed even if guidelines are going to retain a modest role as sources of guidance to clinicians. If they are scripted to have a more central part in management of professional activity and rationing, as envisaged by the National Institute for Clinical Excellence (NICE), the problems become more serious.

Development

Guideline development refers to the construction of a document that makes recommendations about clinical practice and, within current guideline ideology, links these to research evidence. Problems in the development of primary care guidelines may arise from:

- the resources required to develop high-quality guidelines;
- the nature of the underlying evidence;
- the derivation of recommendations from the evidence.

Resources

The rigour of guideline development is frequently proportional to its cost. Systematic searching for relevant studies, appraising and summarising them, formulating recommendations with balanced development groups and use of external referees are hallmarks of robust guidelines but are expensive. Until 1996, 19 national guidelines[1] in the USA cost between $400,000 and $1 million each. In the UK, costs have been more modest, but even a relatively small guideline can cost up to £60,000 (Waddell *et al.* 1996). At a local level these resources are not available, but that has not stopped the proliferation of *de novo* local guidelines of varying quality. The advent of NICE and the growth of the Scottish Intercollegiate Guidelines Network are welcome, if only because the investment in national guidelines is a more rational use of resources for guidelines development. My concern about NICE-endorsed guidelines is not their central origin *per se*, but the potential *imposition* of these guidelines on clinicians, in general, and on primary care teams, in particular.

Resources will still be needed to adapt national guidelines into local versions that are appropriate to particular geographical and health care settings (Feder *et al.* 1999). Where will these resources come from within primary care? Clinical governance and audit budgets are small and will need to be stretched over the adaptation, dissemination and facilitation of multiple guidelines in addition to numerous other functions.

1 http://text.nlm.nih.gov/ftrs/dbaccess/ahcpr

Another source of funding for adaptation (as well as dissemination and facilitation) is the pharmaceutical industry. The record of drug companies involvement in guidelines is controversial, as I shall discuss further below.

Evidence

A distinguishing feature of guidance to clinicians in the form of guidelines is the explicit linking of recommendations to clinical research evidence. The nature of this evidence and its application to decisions about individual patients are hotly debated topics, spawning sharply penned papers (Miles *et al.* 1997, 1998, 1999) and whole journal issues devoted to the controversy (Miles 1999). Here I will side-step the debate about the status and applicability of different forms of research to clinical practice and accept that well-designed randomised controlled trials (RCTs) are the least biased method of testing the effect of a treatment on patients (Jadad *et al.* 1996), even if the application of the evidence to individual patients is complex. I will address three lower-order problems about clinical trial evidence in relation to primary care guidelines:

- the shortage of good-quality trials;
- the setting of most trials;
- the difficulty in moving from evidence to recommendations even when the nature of the evidence is not contested.

The majority of treatment trials compare single agents against placebo with highly selected patient populations and are often underpowered and poorly designed. In their review of the quality of published drug studies, Bero & Rennie (1996) found that the majority of studies suffered from poor monitoring, poor analysis, illogical conclusions and probable publication bias. They highlighted the disappointing quality of many trials funded by the pharmaceutical industry. Trials of questionable quality are not only a problem in the evaluation of drug therapy: trial methodology is even weaker in the evaluation of other interventions, such as, for example, physical therapy in the management of back pain (Bouler *et al.* 1998). As well as poor-quality trials, there is great paucity of RCTs for many conditions and treatment decisions, making it difficult to come to any conclusion about the effect of specific interventions. The choice of interventions is also influenced by the availability of funding. When assessing the evidence for pain management for acute back pain guidelines, I was struck by the preponderance of trials for new anti-inflammatories and the small number of trials with simple analgesics (van Tulder *et al.* 1998); this imbalance clearly reflects the priorities of the companies funding the trials. Whole categories of intervention, such as complementary therapies, may be relatively neglected, owing to a combination of therapist suspicion of trial methodology and the absence of funding. This results in an absence of evidence for potentially useful treatments, about which guidelines therefore have to remain silent.

The shortage of relevant trials is striking even in well-researched areas like coronary heart disease. Only 62 per cent of the recommendations made in the North of England angina guidelines (North of England Evidence-Based Guideline Development Project 1996) were based on RCTs or meta-analyses. The proportion will be even lower with other conditions. If RCTs are the bedrock on which treatment recommendations are made, all guidelines in the conceivable future will have large areas with recommendations built on less solid ground. A virtue of evidence-based guidelines is their transparency, but this does not reduce the patchy nature of the evidence on which they are based.

Can systematic reviews compensate for the variable quality and small sample sizes of many trials? In principle, systematic reviews or meta-analyses should support both the synthesis of evidence and the development of guidelines. Most systematic reviews now incorporate explicit appraisal of the quality of studies and, by combining the data in meta-analyses, are not limited by the sample sizes of individual studies. The canonical case for the usefulness of meta-analysis is that for streptokinase treatment for acute myocardial infarction. Antman *et al.* (1992) showed, retrospectively, that by 1977 small trials of streptokinase administered during acute myocardial infarction, if combined in a meta-analysis, had shown a significant fall in mortality. It took another ten years and two 'mega trials' (GISSI and ISIS-2) before thrombolysis became standard practice. However, there are cautionary counter-examples, such as the administration of magnesium after myocardial infarction, where seven trials, when combined, showed a substantial fall in mortality by 1990, and magnesium was recommended as an 'effective, safe, simple and inexpensive intervention' in 1993 from an updated meta-analysis. When ISIS-4 data were added to the analysis, the effect on mortality was no longer significant, with the previously positive result probably due to publication bias (Egger & Smith 1995). Administration of magnesium post-myocardial infarction may still give guideline developers a headache, as proponents of magnesium argue that the meta-analysis is misleading (Seelig *et al.* 1998). The sentinel role of meta-analysis is further cast into doubt by Lelorier *et al.*'s study (1997) of the outcomes of 12 large RCTs. They found that the main results of the trials had not been predicted accurately 35 per cent of the time by the meta-analyses published previously on the same topics.

Systematic reviews, either pre-existing or commissioned for guidelines development, are still valuable for making sense of clinical research evidence, but cannot necessarily resolve differences between trials of the same intervention. The potential confusion for guideline developers has grown as the systematic review industry moves into high gear. 'Discordant' reviews and meta-analyses from different groups have now emerged (Jadad *et al.* 1997).

If there is a shortage of RCTs in general, trials based in primary care are in even shorter supply. Interventions that are administered in secondary care research clinics in a highly selected group of patients may not have the same effect in general practice. For example, the evidence for effective primary prevention of stroke in patients with atrial fibrillation is based on trials with relatively fit older patients monitored in hospital clinics (Atrial Fibrillation Investigators 1994). How applicable is this evidence to the patients with atrial fibrillation I see in my surgery or on home visits? The absolute number of primary-care-based trials is small. Silagy (1993) managed to find only 287 RCTs relevant to primary care in a MEDLINE search over a three-year period (1987–91). The NHS R&D programme, the Medical Research Council and major charities are trying to address this shortcoming by funding pragmatic primary-care-based trials, but for the conceivable future the majority of RCTs will be in other settings. Primary care guideline developers constantly need to interpolate or extrapolate evidence generated in other contexts, which increases the uncertainty of guideline recommendations.

Making recommendations from research evidence – the main aim of guidelines – is not a mechanical process. Recommendations do not emerge spontaneously from the evidence and not only for the reasons discussed above, shortage of relevant trials with consistent results based in primary care. Recommendations always require judgement and consensus on the part of development groups. The composition of these groups and the identity of external referees will influence final recommendations. Guidelines derived from similar evidence may result in substantially different recommendations. Fahey & Peters (1996) analysed the recommendations of five contemporary hypertension guidelines and applied them to 876 patients with diagnosed hypertension on antihypertensive treatment. They found that the proportion of patients with controlled hypertension varied from 17.5 to 84.6 per cent with the different guidelines after adjustment for the sampling method. More recent versions of these guidelines continue to differ (Psaty & Furberg 1999), with conflicting lists of special circumstances when standard antihypertensive treatment is not appropriate. These guidelines had originated from different countries and may therefore reflect cultural differences in medical practice or the varying influence of pharmaceutical companies. Cultural differences may also account for variation in breast and ovarian cancer treatment guidelines in France and the USA (Eisinger *et al.* 1999). Variations in the recommendations of evidence-based guidelines on the same conditions highlight the conditional and consensual nature of these texts.

Dissemination

Even if a robust development process minimises the problems highlighted above, guidelines will not have an effect on clinical practice unless they are brought to the attention of clinicians. Dissemination is a pre-requisite for implementation and a number of obstacles need to be addressed, such as: conflicting guidelines on the same condition; poor-quality, biased guidelines; many guidelines on different conditions; and resources for dissemination/facilitation. The development or 'kite-marking' of primary care guidelines by NICE will not automatically overcome these obstacles.

In a survey of coronary heart disease guidelines (Cluzeau *et al.* 1999) we found 33 guidelines in one region and 205 nationally. Recommendations in these guidelines may conflict, undermining their credibility for clinicians. The problem is compounded by the poor quality of many guidelines, either from lack of resources to develop evidence-based versions or because of their use subtly to market drugs, either through increasing volume of a class of drugs or promotion of a particular brand. For example, dyspepsia guidelines published with an 'educational grant' from Astra Pharmaceuticals gave pride of place to that company's own proton pump inhibitor.

In principle, the introduction of NICE guidelines will address these two obstacles to dissemination. National guidelines have the potential to rise above the clamour of conflicting guidelines from different sources. If they are developed with sound methods, reducing bias and open to external scrutiny, then they are more likely to be noticed and consulted by practising clinicians. By necessity, NICE will have to retain the support of relevant bodies, like the Royal Colleges and professional societies, which have both a leading role in guidelines development and political clout. Although awareness of NICE guidelines will be enhanced by their 'national' status and the support of powerful professional bodies, this does not necessarily confer validity. Recommendations will still be open to challenge on scientific and policy grounds and the existence of other national and international guidelines with different recommendations will always make dissemination complex.

The sheer number of guidelines targeted at general practitioners will remain a problem even with the dissemination of NICE guidelines. Of the 13 topics on which NICE plans to give guidance in the coming year, six are directly relevant to general practice. In addition to guidance on these specific treatments, the present year will see the emergence of national service frameworks introduced and monitored by the Commission for Health Improvement (CHI). My own experience suggests that it is unrealistic to disseminate more than two guidelines a year covering important conditions and requiring change or reorganisation of practice. The current discourse of NICE and the link to review criteria or national standard-setting do not seem to acknowledge that there are limitations on what practices can absorb.

National dissemination of guidelines is generally not effective nor is 'passive' dissemination (i.e. publishing guidelines in journals or sending them directly to clinicians) (Feder *et al.* 1999). Active dissemination or facilitation (Mott *et al.* 1998) will be essential for a wide range of guidelines, and will be expensive in primary care, particularly if practice-based educational methods are employed. Where is the budget for this activity going to come from? As mentioned above, clinical governance budgets are not generous. Although it is conceivable that guideline dissemination can be yoked to educational programmes and continuing professional development, this will depend on general practitioners and nurses in primary care prioritising this over other educational objectives. These challenges to effective dissemination are not unique to national guidelines, but if the status of guidelines changes from guidance to the underpinning of regulatory action, then the lack of investment in dissemination programmes becomes more controversial. The widespread suspicion about guidelines among doctors has partly abated, but will come roaring back if they are converted into financial targets.

Implementation

If, despite all the obstacles, good-quality guidelines are effectively disseminated to doctors and nurses in primary care, guidelines may still fail to have a positive effect on day-to-day clinical practice because of poor implementation. Three problematic aspects of implementation in primary care are worth considering:

- local resources/facilities;
- integration into clinical decision-making;
- wider task of general practitioner.

Local resources/facilities

The problem of limited resources in relation to clinical guidelines does not end with the cost of development (or adaptation) and dissemination. The recommendations contained in guidelines will have direct resource implications for primary care groups and individual clinicians. This is because recommendations will directly affect the prescribing budget that is now cash-limited at the level of the primary care group. For example, recommendations about the prescribing of statins to patients at high risk of myocardial (re-)infarction will increase drug expenditure. Even if this is ultimately cost-effective, because it reduces hospital admissions, there are no mechanisms for shifting resources between prescribing and commissioning budgets. Guidelines at present, and in the conceivable future, do not address cost-effectiveness. In any case, the value judgements that underpin economic analyses of clinical interventions are debatable. These dilemmas are not exclusive to guidelines, but they do contribute to the contingent nature of guidelines and, again, cast doubt on their role as regulatory documents rather than guidance.

Other examples from my own experience of wrestling with the resource implications of guidelines implementation include: (i) absence of an *H. pylori* testing service in one locality in east London when this was the cornerstone of management recommendations for younger people in dyspepsia guidelines; (ii) long waiting-lists for MRI scan when quick access for patients with persistent radiculopathy is a key recommendation in back pain guidelines; (iii) the long waiting-list for angiography when this is the main procedure for coronary heart disease patients for whom revascularisation might be appropriate. Well-developed evidence-based guidelines may support arguments for more resources. But the absolute shortfall in resources introduces another obstacle to full implementation of guidelines, over and above the ignoring of (or resistance to) recommendations by clinicians.

Integration into clinical decision-making

Implementation of specific guidelines is challenging, even if extra resources are not required. How guidelines influence clinical policy or decisions is not well understood. There is relatively little research about decision-making in primary care consultations, although the consultation itself has been closely scrutinised and conceptualised as a key activity in general practice (Ram *et al.* 1999). Clinical decision-making in general is criticised for errors in diagnosis and treatment. Champions of electronic decision support systems linked to individual patient data argue that this is the future for clinical guidelines. Our understanding of the heuristics of clinical practice and how paper-based, 'passive' guidelines are actually used lags far behind this aspiration.

Although decision-making in the consultation is still largely a 'black box', we have some trial evidence about how to promote implementation from trials of guidelines. Patient-specific reminders embedded in patient records to highlight guideline recommendations during consultations are more effective than general reminders about the existence of guidelines or general audit and feedback (Grimshaw & Russell 1993). There is a disjunction between guidelines that have a role in continuing professional development as source documents about evidence-based practice and guidelines that are applied in decisions about or with individual patients. Electronic medical records and formal decision support methods give the technical means for guidelines to be used in the 'real time' of the consultation.

A recently updated review of computerised clinical decision support systems concluded that these systems can improve clinician performance (Hunt *et al.* 1998). But, as Delaney *et al.* (1999, p.1281) point out, they have not lived up to their potential in primary care settings 'on account of a failure to examine the needs of practitioners adequately'. These authors also point to the danger that 'increasing technology will reduce rather than enhance the patient centred nature of data'. It is too early to tell whether this danger will be realised and there are some reasons to think that electronic guidelines may support *greater* involvement of patients in decision-making if they are based on individual estimates of risk and benefit. The use of individual patient absolute risk is an important development in guidelines, particularly in cardiovascular medicine. The recently published national coronary heart disease guidelines include risk tables linked to treatment recommendations. This necessarily takes the guidelines directly into the consultation and increases their effect on clinical decisions and, if the data and decisions are shared with the patient, on shared decision-making.

The potential of electronic guidelines to improve the quality of clinical decisions and patient involvement is unarguable. But the same technology that brings the guidelines into the consultation can contribute to their imposition on clinicians. The micro-regulation of clinical practice by managed care programmes in the USA demonstrates how patient data and the recording of diagnostic and treatment decisions allow external control and regulation. The regulatory function of NICE and CHI, mediated by the clinical governance responsibilities of primary care groups, can encompass individual clinician behaviour with these data. As a researcher into guidelines implementation, I am enthusiastic about enhancing guidelines use and patient partnership through the use of electronic guidelines and decision support. As a clinician, I am wary about the control over clinical decisions moving *outside* the consultation. Yet even within the consultation, the role of guidelines may be problematic, as the consultation is not only a context for 'rational' decision-making, but also 'the patient's forum for coming to understand her illness' (Toon 1994).

The GP–patient relationship

So, let us finally turn to a deeper level of concern about the use of guidelines in primary care, a concern that will be amplified many-fold if national guidelines become regulatory instruments. The relationship over time between general practitioner and patient addresses a central need for people with chronic or recurrent illness: a search for meaning. Iona Heath (1995, p.19) expresses this eloquently in a monograph on the *Mystery of General Practice*:

> 'The general practitioner, often seeing patients through twenty or thirty years of illness and disease, both major and minor, as well as a series of significant life events, is in a unique position to help the patient make some sense of what is happening to them ... The doctor witnesses the suffering, the struggle and the fortitude of the patient and the relationship is one of solidarity. The patient is allowed and enabled to tell the story of their illness to the doctor during a succession of consultations which may extend over many years.'

The growing emphasis on guidelines and clinical decision-making may marginalise this hermeneutic role of the general practitioner. This is speculative, although there is evidence that the use of a computer in consultation is associated with an increase in topics raised by the doctor and a reduction in those raised by the patient (Pringle *et al.* 1995).

In terms of quality assurance, guidelines, as they are presently constituted, are a manifestation of an absolutist definition of quality. The aggressive implementation of such guidelines may create a new barrier between clinician and patient. If we are genuinely seeking a more equal relationship with patients based on partnership rather than paternalism, guidelines could present a problem unless we find satisfactory ways of sharing recommendations and also rationing their use, to prevent them, rather than the patient, dictating the form and content of the consultation.

Conclusion

By outlining conceptual and methodological problems with primary care guidelines in their development, dissemination and implementation, I have arrived at a simple conclusion: guidelines are crude and fragile instruments. Crude, because of the quality of the underlying evidence and the consensual construction of recommendations. Fragile, because they can quickly lose credibility when applied to the problems of individual patients, or because there are insufficient local resources to implement them.

I remain convinced that robustly developed guidelines with well-designed implementation have the potential to improve the quality of primary care. The dangers that guidelines pose to the broader goals of general practice are real, but can be diffused if they remain sources of guidance and do not become the basis of professional regulation. To date, press releases from NICE have emphasised guidance, but standard-setting is part of the Institute's remit, and CHI has an explicit quality assurance and regulatory function. We need to ensure that the complex and uncertain relationship between guidelines and clinical practice is not forgotten in a political climate that appears determined to achieve professional regulation and control.

Acknowledgements

The ideas in this chapter have their origins in discussion and collaboration with Allen Hutchinson, Richard Baker, Martin Eccles, Chris Griffiths, Jeremy Grimshaw and Brian Hurwitz.

References

Antman EM, Lau J, Kupelnick B, Mosteller F & Chalmers TC (1992). A comparison of results of meta-analyses of randomized control trials and recommendations of clinical experts. Treatments for myocardial infarction. *JAMA* **268**, 240–8.

Atrial Fibrillation Investigators (1994). Risk factors for stroke and efficacy of anti-thrombotic therapy in atrial fibrillation: analysis of pooled data from five randomized trials. *Arch Intern Med* **154**, 1449–57.

Bero LA & Rennie D (1996). Influences on the quality of published drug studies [Review] [146 refs]. *Int J Technol Assess Health Care* **12**, 209–37.

Bouter LM, van Tulder MW & Koes BW (1998). Methodologic issues in low back pain research in primary care. *Spine* **23**, 2014–20.

Cluzeau F, Littlejohns P, Grimshaw J & Feder G (1997). National survey of UK clinical guidelines for the management of coronary heart disease, lung and breast cancer, asthma and depression. *J Clin Effect* **2**,120–4

Cluzeau F, Littlejohns P, Grimshaw J, Feder G & Moran S (1999). Development and application of a generic methodology to assess the quality of clinical guidelines. *Int J for Quality in Health Care* **11**, 21–8.

Delaney BC, Fitzmaurice DA, Riaz A & Hobbs FD (1999). Can computerised decision support systems deliver improved quality in primary care? *BMJ* **319**, 1281.

Egger M & Smith GD (1995). Misleading meta-analysis. *BMJ* **310**, 752–4.

Eisinger F, Geller G, Burke W & Holtzman NA (1999). Cultural basis for differences between US and French clinical recommendations for women at increased risk of breast and ovarian cancer. *Lancet* **353**, 919–20.

Fahey TP & Peters TJ (1996). What constitutes controlled hypertension? Patient based comparison of hypertension guidelines [see comments]. *BMJ* **313**, 93–6.

Feder G, Griffiths C, Highton C, Eldridge S, Spence M & Southgate L (1995). Do clinical guidelines introduced with practice based education improve care of asthmatic and diabetic patients? A randomised controlled trial in general practices in east London. *BMJ* **311**, 1473–8.

Feder G, Eccles M, Grol R, Griffiths C & Grimshaw J (1999). Clinical guidelines: using clinical guidelines. *BMJ* **318**, 728–30.

Field M & Lohr KN (1992). Guidelines for clinical practice: from development to use. *BMJ* **311**, 370–3.

Grimshaw JM & Russell IT (1993). Effect of clinical guidelines on medical practice: a systematic review of rigorous evaluations. *Lancet* **342**, 1317–22.

Heath I (1995). The mystery of general practice. Nuffield Provincial Hospital Trust, London.

Hunt DL, Haynes RB, Hanna SE & Smith K (1998). Effects of computer-based clinical decision support systems on physician performance and patient outcomes: a systematic review [see comments]. *JAMA* **280**, 1339–46.

Jadad AR, Moore RA, Carroll D *et al.* (1996). Assessing the quality of reports of randomized clinical trials: is blinding necessary? *Controlled Clin Trials* **17**, 1–12.

Jadad AR, Cook DJ & Browman GP (1997). A guide to interpreting discordant systematic reviews. *CMAJ* **156**, 1411–16.

LeLorier J, Gregoire G, Benhaddad A, Lapierre J & Derderian F (1998). Discrepancies between meta-analyses and subsequent large randomized, controlled trials [see comments]. *N Engl J Med* **337**, 536–42.

Littlejohns P, Cluzeau F, Bale R, Grimshaw J, Feder G & Moran S (1999). The quantity and quality of clinical practice guidelines for the management of depression in primary care in the UK [in process citation]. *Br J Gen Pract* **49**, 205–10.

Majno G (1975). *The healing hand: man and wound in the ancient world.* Harvard University Press, Cambridge (Mass.), USA.

Miles A (ed.) (1999). Advancing the evidence-based health care debate [Thematic edition]. *J Eval Clin Pract* **5**, 97–263.

Miles A, Bentley P, Polychronis A & Grey J (1997). Evidence-based medicine. Why all the fuss? This is why. *Journal of Evaluation in Clinical Practice* **3**, 83–6.

Miles A, Bentley P, Polychronis A, Grey J & Price N (1998). Recent progress in health services research: on the need for evidence-based debate. *Journal of Evaluation in Clinical Practice* **4**, 257–65.

Miles A, Bentley P, Polychronis A, Grey J & Price N (1999). Advancing the evidence-based healthcare debate. *Journal of Evaluation in Clinical Practice* **5**, 97–101.

Mott S, Feder G, Griffiths C & Donovan S (1998). Coronary heart disease in general practice guidelines. Practice based audit: results from a dissemination and implementation programme. *J Clin Effect* **3**, 1–4.

North of England Evidence-Based Guideline Development Project (1996). *Evidence based clinical practice guideline: the primary care management of stable angina.* Centre for Health Services Research, University of Newcastle-upon-Tyne, Newcastle-upon-Tyne.

Pringle M, Dixon P, Carr-Hill R & Ashworth A (1995). *Influences on computer use in general practice. Report of a one-year study on behalf of the Royal College of General Practitioners.* Occasional Paper 68. Royal College of General Practitioners, Exeter.

Psaty BM & Furberg CD (1999). British guidelines on managing hypertension. Provide evidence, progress, and an occasional missed opportunity. *BMJ* **319**, 589–90.

Seelig MS, Elin RJ & Antman EM (1998). Magnesium in acute myocardial infarction: still an open question. *Can J Cardiol* **14**, 745–9.

Ram P, Grol R, Rethans JJ, Schouten B, van d V & Kester A (1999). Assessment of general practitioners by video observation of communicative and medical performance in daily practice: issues of validity, reliability and feasibility. *Med Educ* **33**, 447–54.

Silagy C (1993). Developing a register of randomised controlled trials in primary care [published erratum appears in *BMJ* 1993; **306**:1660] [see comments]. *BMJ* **306**, 897–900.

Sweeney K (1996). Evidence and uncertainty. In *Sense and sensibility in health care* (ed. M Marinker), pp.59–87. London, BMJ Publishing Group.

Toon P (1994). *What is good general practice?* Occasional Paper 65. Royal College of General Practitioners, Exeter.

van Tulder MW, Koes BW & Bouter LM (1998). Conservative treatment of acute and chronic nonspecific low back pain: a systematic review of randomized controlled trials of the most common interventions. *Spine* **22**, 2128–56.

Waddell G, Feder G, McIntosh A, Lewis M & Hutchinson A (1996). Low back pain clinical guidelines and evidence review. Royal College of General Practitioners, London.

Woolf SH, Grol R, Hutchinson A, Eccles M & Grimshaw J (1999). Clinical guidelines: potential benefits, limitations, and harms of clinical guidelines. *BMJ* **318**, 527–30.

Chapter 5

Evidence, guidelines, audit and cardiology: principles and problems in secondary and tertiary care

John R Hampton

Introduction

'The end of clinical freedom' was announced, without regret, in a *British Medical Journal* editorial in 1983 (Hampton 1983). It was suggested that doctors had to abandon their time-honoured 'right' to do what they regarded as 'the best' for their individual patients. This had become necessary for two reasons. First, increasing evidence of which treatments were effective and which were not was accumulating from randomised clinical trials. Some 30 years after the first clinical trial which meets modern requirements – the MRC trial of streptomycin in tuberculosis (MRC 1948) – the unreliability of an individual doctor's expertise and opinion was beginning to be accepted, and the need for adequate clinical trials had become a routine part of the medical ethos. Second, increasing possibilities in medical care had apparently reached the limit of what many health care systems were prepared to pay for. Doctors' freedom was therefore going to be financially limited, and especially so if there was no good evidence for the treatment that they recommended. The term 'evidence-based medicine' had not yet been coined in 1983, but now it has certainly supplanted 'clinical freedom' as a medical mantra.

Cardiology has been at the forefront of the development of the philosophy of evidence-based medicine. The statistical problems of clinical trial design and analysis had for a long time been understood by statisticians, and cardiologists were probably the first clinicians to learn about them and design trials accordingly. This was perhaps the result of two elements: the high prevalence of cardiovascular disease, and the fact that the pharmaceutical industry was prepared to invest large sums of money in the development of new cardiovascular products because the potential market for them was large. As a result, we have a good 'evidence base' for the management of virtually all cardiovascular problems – from the prevention and treatment of myocardial infarction, the treatment of angina, hypertension, heart failure, venous thrombosis, to arrhythmias.

The safety and efficacy of new drug treatments are assessed by the Medical Control Agency (MCA) and of new devices (pacemakers, defibrillators) by the Medical Devices Agency (MDA). There is no similar body that 'controls' the introduction of new surgical techniques, but it is now accepted that these have to be subjected where possible to clinical trials as much as new drugs, and on the basis of trial evidence purchasers can decide, together with clinicians, whether a new surgical technique should be introduced or not.

What, then, is the potential value of the National Institute for Clinical Excellence (NICE) in cardiology? Is it to tell cardiologists what they already know – what the clinical trials show? Is it to advise purchasers about which MCA-approved treatments are cost-effective? Is the role of NICE to join the myriad of international, national and local bodies, which already produce innumerable guidelines? If NICE disagrees with guidelines for some cardiovascular treatments put out by a body such as the European Society for Cardiology, what should cardiologists believe?

The problem for cardiologists is not a lack of evidence. The problem – funding apart – is the interpretation of the evidence. Does NICE have any better view of the 'truth' than cardiologists who are, after all, specialists in their field? Starting with clinical trials, the difficulty cardiologists have can be considered under three main headings:

- evidence-based medicine;
- opinion-based medicine;
- real-world medicine.

We need to understand where one merges into the other, and to appreciate the limits of practising truly evidence-based medicine. Only then can we decide whether NICE is likely to be helpful.

Evidence-based medicine

There is evidence from clinical trials, most of it very good, that guides the treatment of all the important cardiovascular diseases.

For primary prevention, we know that blood pressure control is important, and a series of studies over two decades or more has shown that the lower the blood pressure, the better (MRC Working Party 1985; Hansson *et al.* 1995). So many different hypotensive agents have been used in different trials that we can be confident that it is blood pressure control that matters, not the way this is achieved. We also have good evidence that reduction of the plasma cholesterol by pravastatin prolongs survival (Shepherd 1995). There is no clinical trial evidence of the benefit of stopping smoking, but the epidemiological evidence is so strong and the non-cardiovascular diseases related to smoking are so important, that further evidence is unnecessary.

In patients with acute myocardial infarction we know that treatment with a variety of thrombolytic agents reduces fatality (ISIS-2 1988; Wilcox *et al.* 1990; INJECT 1995; GUSTO IIb 1997). We know that nitrate treatment is ineffective (ISIS-4 1995). We know that intravenous beta-blockade has an effect in some people (MIAMI 1985; ISIS-1 1986), but later I shall point out deficiencies in the evidence.

Box 5.1 Acronyms of trials referred to in this chapter

BHAT	Beta-blocker Heart Attack Trial
CAMIAT	Canadian Amiodarone Myocardial Infarction Arrhythmia Trial
CAST	Cardiac Arrhythmia Suppression Trial
COBALT	Continuous Infusion Versus Double-Blind Administration of Alteplase
CONSENSUS	Cooperative North Scandinavian Enalapril Survival Study
EMIAT	European Myocardial Infarction Amiodarone Trial
GISSI	Gruppo Italiano per lo Studio della Streptochinasi nell'Infarto Miocardico
GUSTO	Global Use of Strategies to Open Occluded Coronary Arteries
INJECT	International Joint Efficacy Comparison of Thrombolytics
ISIS	International Study of Infarct Survival
MIAMI	Metoprolol in Acute Myocardial Infarction
PACK	Prevention of Atherosclerotic Complications with Ketanserin
RITA	Randomised Intervention Treatment of Angina
SWORD	Survival with oral d-sotalol
TRACE	Trandolapril Cardiac Evaluation Study
TRENT	Trial of Early Nifedipine Treatment

Following myocardial infarction there is excellent evidence of the value of aspirin (Antiplatelet Trialists' Collaboration 1994), beta-blockers (The Norwegian Multicenter Study Group 1981), statins (Scandinavian Simvastatin Survival Study Group 1994; Sacks *et al.* 1996), and angiotensin converting enzyme (ACE) inhibitors (AIRE 1993; Kober *et al.* 1995).

For patients with atrial fibrillation the value of warfarin is unquestionable, and we know about the relative efficacy of warfarin and aspirin (Petersen *et al.* 1989; Veterans Affairs Stroke Prevention 1992; Stroke Prevention in Atrial Fibrillation Investigators 1994).

The evidence base for non-drug treatments is not so secure, partly because interventional techniques advance so rapidly that the results of a trial tend to be out of date before they are published. We know that coronary artery bypass grafting (CABG) and percutaneous transluminal coronary angioplasty (PTCA) are the best ways of relieving angina, and we are reasonably confident that CABG leads to the best survival in patients with certain patterns of vascular disease. The place of PTCA is less securely underpinned by clinical trials: it is excellent for angina relief, and some believe that it produces optimal survival in acute myocardial infarction and unstable angina – but here experts still disagree (RITA-2 1976; European Coronary Surgery Study Group 1982; CASS 1984; RITA Trial Participants 1993; Henderson *et al.* 1998).

This list could be prolonged, but there seem to be enough instances here on which to base guidelines for the treatment of most patients with vascular disease.

Who should have the responsibility to write these guidelines is a problem to discuss when we have considered the limitations of all this excellent evidence.

Cardiology has learned – often the hard way – that 'surrogate' endpoints in clinical trials can be misleading. For example, it was for a long time thought that, since many patients with coronary disease die of ventricular arrhythmias, prevention of these arrhythmias 'made sense'. Several drugs, particularly the Class I anti-arrhythmic drugs, were shown to be effective anti-arrhythmic agents. They were widely used in patients with coronary disease on the assumption that death rates would be reduced. The CAST trial of flecainide and encainide eventually showed that this was not the case and that treatment with these drugs actually increased fatality (CAST 1989). It was then appreciated that drugs of this type were actually pro-arrhythmic, as well as being anti-arrhythmic. It has been suggested that inappropriate use of anti-arrhythmic drugs before the publication of the CAST trial killed more Americans than the Vietnam war.

Once we had CAST, we did not need a National Institute for Clinical Excellence to point out the evident fallacy in the original reason for using anti-arrhythmic drugs. An unusually percipient institute might have given a warning before CAST was published, but this would have been completely contrary to the perceived wisdom of the day. There seems no reason to suppose that a view from a non-specialist institute would materially have affected the behaviour of cardiologists.

The CAST result raised the general question whether all anti-arrhythmic drugs might increase the death rate in patients with coronary disease. This question, applied to other treatments for other vascular diseases, is one of the major general questions that cardiologists now have to answer.

Specifically concerning arrhythmias, it does seem that all Class I anti-arrhythmic agents may, under certain (not always identifiable) circumstances, have undesirable effects: 'quinidine syncope' was, after all, known to exist from the earliest stages of cardiology. It was hoped that the Class III anti-arrhythmic drugs would prolong life by preventing significant arrhythmias, but the SWORD trial of sotalol showed that this was not the case, active treatment being associated with increased fatality (Waldo *et al.* 1996). Only amiodarone seems to reduce deaths due to arrhythmias (the EMIAT and CAMIAT trials) (Schwartz *et al.* 1994; Cairns *et al.* 1997), but amiodarone treatment does not seem to reduce total fatality.

It is thus clear that we cannot group all anti-arrhythmics together as a 'drug class', and each has to be considered separately according to the evidence available. Is this true of other drug types used in different disease states? The answer to this question has major implications for the production of guidelines, and therefore for the activities of NICE.

Opinion-based medicine

ACE inhibitors perhaps provide the best example of a class of drugs, which in their main effects are interchangeable. Different drugs of this type have consistently produced survival benefit in patients with heart failure. Large scale trials with death as an endpoint have been conducted with captopril, enalapril, ramipril and trandolapril (Cohn *et al.* 1991; CONSENSUS 1991; Pfeffer *et al.* 1991, 1992; SOLVD 1992; AIRE 1993; Kober *et al.* 1995). Patients included were those with severe or mild chronic heart failure, heart failure following myocardial infarction, or those with impaired left ventricular function demonstrated by a variety of techniques. Only in one trial (CONSENSUS 2) did the patients treated with an ACE inhibitor fail to derive any benefit (Swedberg *et al.* 1992). It thus seems fair to assume that all patients with heart failure, except some with well-defined contra-indications, should be treated with an ACE inhibitor and it probably does not matter which. This can probably be extended to the ACE inhibitors, such as parindopril, which are widely used but which have not been selected for a major clinical trial with death as an endpoint. Is this a decision that can be taken by an individual physician, or group of physicians, or must we wait for a pronouncement from some 'superior' body such as NICE? We can see here that there is excellent evidence of a class effect for the value of ACE inhibitors, but even so, when it comes to practical therapeutics, there are differences of opinion.

The issue of the class effect was first debated in the 1980s after a long series of trials of the effect of beta-blockers on the survivors of myocardial infarction. Early treatment did not seem to have a marked or convincing benefit, but late treatment (48 hours or more after myocardial infarction) certainly did (Figure 5.1). Most of the trials were too small, and the confidence intervals surrounding the results were therefore too wide, to give unequivocal results. The first such trial to demonstrate significant benefits was that of timolol (The Norwegian Multicenter Study Group 1981). Propranolol was certainly beneficial but in the definitive trial – BHAT – the dosage regimen was complicated and not easy to follow (BHAT 1982). Acebutalol led to a convincing result in fatality (Boisell *et al.* 1990), but by the time that trial was published, interest in beta-blockers had waned and at least in the UK acebutalol is now hardly used. In the UK the two beta-blockers most commonly used for secondary prevention are timolol and atenolol, although atenolol does not figure in the later-treatment post-infarction trials. Evidently there is a general belief that beta-blockers are interchangeable – but Figure 5.1 shows that this may not be so because oxprenolol seems to have been notably ineffective.

The proliferation of trials of different drugs within a class in patients with a common problem – in this case, myocardial infarction – arose because of the desire of each manufacturer to promote a particular product. The problem has left some doubt, not only about the comparability of drugs, but about the appropriate doses. This may be a situation when the best solution is for the clinician to 'follow the trials'. Does this imply, however, that an institute such as NICE should always advise the use of one or two drugs in particular doses? This would lay it open to charge of bias from the pharmaceutical industry. There is no evidence other than that generated

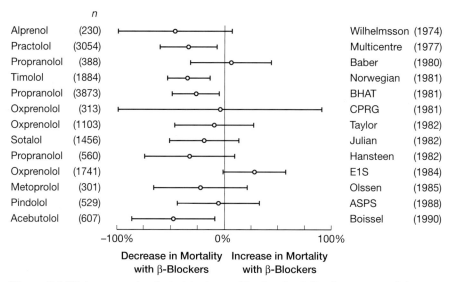

Figure 5.1 Trials comparing beta-blockers with placebo following myocardial infarction, treatment being started 48 hours or more after the onset of symptoms. Horizontal bars show the point estimate for the result with the 95 per cent confidence interval. *n* indicates total no. of patients included in the trial. (For a full list of references see Freemantle *et al.* 1999)

15 or more years ago, so would a new body such as NICE look back over old evidence, over-ride current practice, and advise the use of atenolol for secondary prevention?

The class effect problem becomes rather more important if we consider the statins. Here we have a class of drug where trials of different members – particularly simvastatin and pravastatin – have shown survival advantage in the primary and secondary prevention of myocardial infarction. However, the most potent of this class of drugs, atorvastatin, has not been used in a mortality endpoint trial and the cheapest – cerivastatin – has had least exposure in large trials. The purist may say that clinical practice must follow the result of clinical trials, but can we accept that the statins actually have a class effect? If we can, and if there are no drug-specific adverse effects (which there do not appear to be), then there would seem to be no excuse for using any drug but the cheapest. It is evident that the decision about the existence of a class effect is in the end a matter of opinion, and this is where, like it or not, we are practising 'opinion-based medicine'.

The statistical technique of a meta-analysis is based on the belief that trial results from a group of apparently similar drugs can be pooled, and some believe that clinical practice should be based above all on positive results obtained by a meta-analysis of all published information. This is, however, a flawed concept that does not often work out in practice (LeLorier *et al.* 1997).

Meta-analysis is at its best when many trials of a single drug, used to treat a variety of patients, are combined. A consistent answer suggests that the value of the drug has wide applicability. Aspirin makes a good example: there are a few good individual trials and a lot of less good trials, which together make a powerful argument for the use of aspirin in patients with disease in the coronary, cerebral, or peripheral arteries (Antiplatelet Trialists' Collaboration 1994). There remains a problem of what dose to use, but perhaps that can be decided on the basis of individual trials. However, the results of meta-analysis become insecure if trials of different drugs are combined, if the drugs are used in different ways, and if patients are followed for different lengths of time. For example, is it possible to extend the benefit of aspirin to all antiplatelet agents? Some meta-analyses combined aspirin trials with those of other drugs with quite different effects.

The answer to this is clearly 'no'. Ketanserin was an effective antiplatelet agent, acting by a different mechanism from aspirin. A drug-specific effect (prolongation of the QT interval on the ECG) meant that its use could be hazardous. This was only demonstrated when a large mortality endpoint trial – PACK – was conducted (PACK 1989). The new group of antiplatelet agents, the glycoprotein IIb/IIIa receptor antagonists would in theory be more effective than aspirin because they block the 'final common path' of platelet aggregation. In fact, the oral compounds in this group – orbofiban, xemilofiban and sibrafiban – have been found to be ineffective and their development has been abandoned. It is quite clear that there are differences between antiplatelet agents, and their effects must never be evaluated by a common meta-analysis. But what might happen if NICE were dominated by people who believed that clinical practice should be based on this technique?

Despite a wealth of evidence, clinical practice is going to be based to a large extent on the way in which evidence is interpreted. If evidence-based medicine is, in effect, opinion-based medicine, whose opinion is most valuable?

Drug development occasionally produces totally new drug classes – beta-blockers, ACE inhibitors, statins – but much more often new drugs are members of an existing class. The pharmaceutical industry feels it is worth developing such compounds because they may have drug-specific advantages. For example, they may have fewer, or different, unwanted effects. They may be easier to administer. Above all, they may be cheaper than the first drugs of that class to be introduced. It is intrinsically unlikely – particularly if the main action is a class effect – that a new drug within a class will have a major advantage over its predecessors in terms of, say, mortality reduction.

To demonstrate whether one active drug is superior in its main action to a related drug would require a huge study, and the expense is such that few direct comparisons are undertaken. The very large trials comparing two thrombolytics (ISIS-3, GISSI-2) and GUSTO, comparing streptokinase and alteplase, were exceptions (The International Study Group 1990; ISIS-3 1992; GUSTO IIb 1997). But a new drug will be thought worthwhile if it has some specific advantage when its main effect is equivalent to its predecessors. The definition of 'equivalence' has proved difficult, and has shown that even after the application of rigorous statistical principles, opinion is crucial.

Figure 5.2 illustrates the difficulty of defining equivalence. If two drugs A and B are compared, the superiority of one will be demonstrated if the 95 per cent confidence interval around the observed difference in effect (the point estimate) excludes the possibility of zero difference. Thus in the example shown in the top line of Figure 5.2, drug A is clearly superior to drug B. In the second line, drug B is superior. In the example in the third line, there is no difference between the effects of the two drugs and the confidence interval around zero is small, so no one would doubt that the two drugs are equivalent. In the fourth example, there is again no difference in effect, but the confidence interval around zero difference is large: there is thus a real possibility that either drug A or B is superior, and there would be doubt about calling the two equivalent. There would be even more doubt about a trial like the one shown in the fifth line. Drug A appears superior, but the confidence interval extends beyond zero, so the difference is not significant. In this trial, could equivalence be claimed? In the final example, drug A is superior to B with a small confidence interval, but the absolute benefit is small and the difference could be regarded as clinically unimportant.

Figure 5.2 makes it clear that the concept of equivalence has to have a statistical basis – it is necessary to define the acceptable width of the confidence interval around the expected point estimate of the trial result – but in the end, what is equivalent is a matter of judgement. Or, perhaps more accurately, of opinion.

The first major trial designed specifically to demonstrate equivalence was INJECT, a comparison of the thrombolytic agents streptokinase and reteplase in patients with acute myocardial infarction (INJECT 1995). It was decided on pragmatic and clinical grounds that, provided it was reasonably certain that the fatality rate associated with reteplase treatment was no more than 1 per cent greater than that with streptokinase, the drugs could be considered equivalent. This set the limit, but

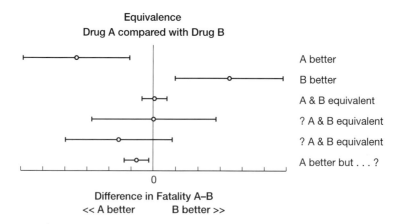

Figure 5.2 Possible results from clinical trials comparing two drugs, A and B. The zero line represents no difference in their effect. Horizontal bars represent the possible point estimates of the results with their confidence intervals

statistical principles were needed to calculate the necessary trial size. On the basis of angiographic studies it was predicted that patients treated with reteplase would have a fatality rate 1 per cent less than those treated with streptokinase. It was calculated that with a trial of about 6,000 patients the objective would be achieved if the fatality rate with reteplase was 0.5 per cent less than that with streptokinase. The confidence interval around such a result would include zero difference, but would fall short of a 1 per cent superiority of reteplase. In the event, the fatality rate in the reteplase group was 9.02 per cent compared with 9.53 per cent in the streptokinase group. The 95 per cent confidence interval was -1.98–0.96 per cent. The trial thus excluded the possibility that the fatality rate with reteplase was 1 per cent worse then it was with streptokinase, and equivalence was proven.

On the basis of the INJECT trial reteplase was licensed by the FDA, and the concept of equivalence trials gained ground. In a trial called COBALT, an attempt was made to demonstrate the equivalence of a continuous infusion and a double bolus of alteplase (COBALT 1997). Seven thousand patients were included; fatality rates were 7.98 and 7.53 per cent respectively. Few clinicians would consider a difference of 0.48 per cent to be of any importance, but because the limit of equivalence was set at 0.4 per cent, the trial failed in its objective and equivalence could not be claimed.

There is evidently a logical difficulty here, and it demonstrates how opinion (? judgement) controls clinical trial design and interpretation, and shows that what sometimes seems to be 'evidence-based medicine' is actually 'opinion-based medicine'. It could be that NICE might have a role here, deciding on the limits within which two drugs could be considered equivalent. But licensing authorities already have a view about this, and so will a doctor treating an individual patient on the basis of published data. It is difficult to see how NICE could fit easily between the two.

Real-world medicine

Strictly speaking, the results of a clinical trial apply only to those patients who were actually included. The unanswered question is always the extent to which trial results apply to patients with the condition under investigation who were not included. This can be approached in two ways – by asking what proportion of potential patients were included in the trial in the participating centres, and by comparing the outcome of the trial with that of patients seen in routine practice.

A register of all potential trial patients should be an essential part of any clinical trial, but registers are seldom kept. When they are, they often show that only a very small proportion of patients were included in the trial. For example, in the RITA-1 trial comparing PTCA and CABG in patients with stable angina, a register of all coronary angiograms in the participating centres showed that only 3 per cent of patients were included in the study (Henderson *et al.* 1995). There are, however, examples of registers showing a relatively high proportion of patients being included – for example, the TRACE study of trandolopril in patients with left ventricular dysfunction after myocardial infarction (Kober *et al.* 1995). When patients excluded from a clinical trial are followed in the same way as the trial patients, it is almost invariably found that their outcome is worse than that of either the treatment or the control groups within the trials. Thus in the TRENT trial comparing nifedipine or placebo in patients with acute myocardial infarction (Wilcox *et al.* 1986), the fatality rate was 6.7 per cent at one month for patients given nifedipine, 6.3 per cent for those given placebo, but 18.2 per cent for the approximately 50 per cent of patients who were registered but, for some reason, not randomised.

Similarly, patients included in a series of thrombolytic trials in Nottingham had a considerably lower fatality rate (24 per cent compared with 37 per cent at four years) than those who were given a thrombolytic but who did not fulfil the admission criteria of the trial. Patients who were not given a thrombolytic at all had an even worse fatality rate of 60 per cent (Brown *et al.* 1999).

Trial registers and the follow-up of non-trial patients demonstrate what is perhaps obvious. The inclusion and exclusion criteria of clinical trials lead to the trials recruiting younger and more mobile patients who can attend follow-up, and patients free of other diseases and who are not being treated with multiple drugs. The results of the trial therefore apply only to these low-risk patients, which makes the application of 'evidence based-medicine' very difficult in the real world.

The first table in the published results of any clinical trial, which shows the baseline characteristics of the included patients, tells much the same story. The patients are relatively young. Trials of acute myocardial infarction usually show average age of just over 60. Trials in heart failure usually include patients of much the same age, which is even more worrying because heart failure is a disease of the elderly. Elderly patients have multiple diseases and take multiple treatments, some of which (for example, non-steroidal anti-inflammatory drugs) interact with treatments such as ACE inhibitors given for heart failure. Elderly patients have difficulty with compliance, and make a clinical trial 'untidy', so they are seldom included.

The results table of a clinical trial also gives a clue as to whether the results can be carried over to the generality of patients. Thus the two 'positive' trials of intravenous beta-blockers in acute myocardial infarction – MIAMI and ISIS-1 – involved patient groups with a hospital fatality rate of 3 or 4 per cent (MIAMI Trial Research Group 1985; ISIS-1 1986). This is so low by comparison with the true overall fatality of acute myocardial infarction patients that the meaning of these trials to the real world is very doubtful (Brown *et al.* 1997).

Perhaps the best example of the difficulty of translating clinical trial results practised in the real world is the use of anticoagulants in chronic atrial fibrillation. It is clear that anticoagulants are superior to aspirin for preventing stroke (Stroke Prevention in Atrial Fibrillation Investigators 1994), and that the major benefit of anticoagulant treatment is seen in old people with structural heart disease. Unfortunately, these are the very people in whom the use of anticoagulants is most difficult. They are immobile, and ensuring safe and adequate anticoagulant control – particularly in the face of complicated and changing concomitant therapy – is difficult. These patients tend to fall, and a broken hip in a patient on warfarin therapy can be disastrous; a subdural haematoma is even worse. In such patients the balance of risks and benefits from anticoagulant treatment is probably completely different from what a clinical trial suggests.

Real-world medicine is therefore not the same as clinical trial medicine; those who produce 'evidence-based' guidelines for treatment must accept the limitations of the evidence they quote.

The role of NICE and guidelines for cardiovascular therapy

It should now be clear that cardiologists do not need a National Institute for Clinical Excellence. There is no shortage of evidence for the efficacy (and in some cases, lack of efficacy) of cardiovascular therapies. However, the interpretation of the evidence is all too often a matter of opinion. When it comes to opinion, presumably the opinion of cardiovascular experts is more enlightening than that of a national body charged with the development of all aspects of clinical evidence. When it comes to the real world, however, it is individual doctors who have to decide whether their individual patient is sufficiently like those from whom the 'evidence base' was developed to make the use of a particular treatment appropriate. The factors that doctors have to take into account are so varied, and often as vague as the glint in a patient's eye, that having a national guideline in their pocket is unlikely to be helpful.

Given the difficulty of interpreting the considerable evidence base of cardiovascular therapy, guidelines are likely to reflect the lowest common level of agreement. Patients who have had a myocardial infarction need aspirin, a beta-blocker, a statin and (maybe) an ACE inhibitor. Patients with heart failure (usually) need an ACE inhibitor. Patients with high cholesterol levels need a statin, although the cholesterol level that should be treated depends on funding, and the funding decision is a local matter. We do not need another level of therapeutic bureaucracy to produce this sort of document.

If NICE is, in fact, a national institute for *cost-effectiveness,* then curiously this may be less of a problem. Deciding whether a treatment is effective is difficult enough, but deciding whether it is cost-effective is very much a value judgement. It has to involve a comparison with other treatments for other diseases, and so with other value judgements. If NICE were to say that statin therapy post-infarction was not to be used in the under-50s (where the risk is very low) or in the over-70s (who may not live long enough to reap the benefit), then this can be argued by politicians, the lay press and patients. Doctors may advise otherwise, but in a socialised system of medical care those who pay the piper call the tune, and it would be one less decision that doctors had to take.

There are already a multitude of guidelines for cardiovascular treatment, most being modifications of others. If NICE were to be asked to give its seal of approval to all of them it could never achieve anything, for it would do nothing other than read a series of documents with minor, and probably unimportant, differences.

There is nothing wrong with the principle of guidelines, but they must be seen to be for the guidance of wise people and for the obedience of fools. Those who claim expertise in a field do not need nanny to tell them how to treat individual patients.

References

AIRE (The Acute Infarction Ramipril Efficacy) Study Investigators (1993). Effect of ramipril on mortality and morbidity of survivors of acute myocardial infarction with clinical evidence of heart failure. *Lancet* **342**, 821–8.

Antiplatelet Trialists' Collaboration (1994). Collaborative overview of randomised trials of antiplatelet therapy. I: prevention of death, myocardial infarction and stroke by prolonged antiplatelet therapy in various categories of patients. *BMJ* **308**, 81–106.

BHAT (Beta-blocker Heart Attack Trial) Research Group (1982). A randomized trial of propranolol in patients with acute myocardial infarction. 1. Mortality results. *JAMA* **247**, 1707–14.

Boisell J-P, Leizorovicz A, Picolet H & Peyrieux J-C, for the APSI Investigators (1990). Secondary prevention after high-risk acute myocardial infarction with low-dose acebutolol. *Am J Cardiol* **66**, 251–60.

Brown N, Melville M, Gray D, Young T, Skene AM, Wilcox RG & Hampton JR (1999). Relevance of clinical trial results in myocardial infarction to medical practice: comparison of four year outcome in participants of a thrombolytic trial, patients receiving routine thrombolysis, and those deemed ineligible for thrombolysis. *Heart* **81**, 598–602.

Brown N, Young T, Gray D, Skene AM & Hampton JR. (1997). Inpatient deaths from acute myocardial infarction, 1982–92: analysis of data in the Nottingham Heart Attack Register. *BMJ* **315**, 159–64.

Cairns JA, Connolly SJ, Roberts R & Gent M, for the Canadian Amiodarone Myocardial Infarction Arrhythmia Trial Investigators (1997). Randomised trial of outcome after myocardial infarction in patients with frequent or repetitive ventricular premature depolarisations: CAMIAT. *Lancet* **349**, 675–82.

CASS Principal Investigators and Their Associates (1984). Myocardial infarction and mortality in the Coronary Artery Surgery Study (CASS) randomised trial. *N Engl J Med* **310**, 7508.

CAST (The Cardiac Arrhythmia Suppression Trial) Investigators (1989). Preliminary report: effect of encainide and flecainide on mortality in a randomized trial of arrhythmia suppression after myocardial infarction. *N Engl J Med* **321**, 406–12.

COBALT (Continuous Infusion versus Double-Blind Administration of Alteplase) Investigators (1997). A comparison of continuous infusion of alteplase with double-bolus administration for acute myocardial infarction. *N Engl J Med* **337**, 1124–30.

Cohn JN, Johnson G, Ziesche S *et al.* (1991) A comparison of enalapril with hydralazine-isosorbide dinitrate in the treatment of chronic congestive heart failure. *N Engl J Med* **325**, 303–10.

CONSENSUS (Cooperative North Scandinavian Enalapril Survival Study) Trial Study Group (1991). Effects of enalapril on mortality in severe congestive heart failure; results of the Cooperative North Scandinavian Enalapril Survival Study (CONSENSUS). *N Engl J Med* **316**, 1429–35.

European Coronary Surgery Study Group (1982). Long-term results of prospective randomised study of coronary artery bypass surgery in stable angina pectoris. *Lancet* **2**, 1174–82.

Freemantle N, Cleland J, Young P, Mason J & Harrison J (1999). β-blockade after myocardial infarction: systematic review and meta regression analysis. *BMJ* **318**, 1730–7.

GUSTO IIb (Global Use of Strategies to Open Occluded Coronary Arteries in Acute Coronary Syndromes) (1997). Angiographic Substudy Investigators. *N Engl J Med* **336**, 1621–8.

Hampton JR (1982). Should every survivor of a heart attack be given a beta-blocker? Part I. Evidence from clinical trials. *Br Med J* **285**, 33–40.

Hampton JR (1983). The end of clinical freedom. *Br Med J* **287**, 1237–8.

Hansson L, Zanchetti A, Carruthers SG *et al.,* for the HOT Study Group (1998). Effects of intensive blood-pressure lowering and low-dose aspirin in patients with hypertension: principal results of the hypertension optimal treatment (HOT) randomised trial. *Lancet* **351**,1755–62.

Henderson RA, Raskino CL & Hampton JR (1995). Variations in the use of coronary arteriograph in the UK: the RITA trial coronary arteriogram register. *Q J Med* **88**, 167–73.

Henderson RA, Pocock SJ, Sharp SJ, Nanchahal K, Sculpher MJ, Buxton MJ, Hampton JR for the Randomised Intervention Treatment of Angina (RITA-1) trial participants (1998). Long-term results of RITA-1 trial: clinical and cost comparisons of coronary angioplasty and coronary artery bypass grafting. *Lancet* **352**, 1419–25.

INJECT (International Joint Efficacy Comparison of Thrombolytics) Trial Study Group (1995). Randomised, double-blind comparison of reteplase double-bolus administration with streptokinase in acute myocardial infarction (INJECT): trial to investigate equivalence. *Lancet* **346**, 329–36.

The International Study Group (1990). In-hospital mortality and clinical course of 20,891 patients with suspected acute myocardial infarction randomised between alteplase and streptokinase with or without heparin. *Lancet* **336**, 71–5.

ISIS-1 (First International Study of Infarct Survival) Collaborative Group (1986). Randomised trial of intravenous atenolol among 16,027 cases of suspected acute myocardial infarction: ISIS-1. *Lancet* **2**, 57–66.

ISIS-2 (Second International Study of Infarct Survival) (1988). Collaborative group randomised trial of intravenous streptokinase, oral aspirin, both or neither among 17,187 cases of suspected acute myocardial infarction: ISIS-2. *Lancet* **2**, 349–60.

ISIS-3 (Third International Study of Infarct Survival) (1992). A randomised trial of streptokinase vs tissue plasminogen activator vs anistreplase and of aspirin plus heparin vs aspirin alone among 41,299 cases of suspected acute myocardial infarction. *Lancet* **339**, 753–70.

ISIS-4 (Fourth International Study of Infarct Survival) Collaborative Group (1995). ISIS-4: A randomised factorial trial assessing early oral captopril, oral mononitrate, and intravenous magnesium sulphate in 58,050 patients with suspected acute myocardial infarction. *Lancet* **345**, 669–85.

Kober L *et al.*, for the Trandolapril Cardiac Evaluation (TRACE) Study Group (1995). A clinical trial of the angiotensin-converting-enzyme inhibitor trandolapril in patients with left ventricular dysfunction after myocardial infarction. *N Engl J Med* **333**, 1670–6.

LeLorier J, Gregoire G, Benhaddad A, Lapierre J & Derderian F (1997). Discrepancies between meta-analyses and subsequent large randomised, controlled trials. *N Engl J Med* **337**, 536–42.

MIAMI (Metoprolol in Acute Myocardial Infarction) Trial Research Group (1985). Metoprolol in acute myocardial infarction (MIAMI). A randomised placebo-controlled international trial. *European Heart Journal* **6**, 199–226.

[MRC] Medical Research Council Investigation (1948). Streptomycin treatment of pulmonary tuberculosis. *Br Med J* **2**, 669–782.

[MRC] Medical Research Council Working Party (1985). MRC trial of treatment of mild hypertension: principal results. *Br Med J* **291**, 97–104.

The Norwegian Multicenter Study Group (1981). Timolol-induced reduction in mortality and reinfarction in patients surviving acute myocardial infarction. *N Engl J Med* **304**, 801–7.

Petersen P, Boysen G, Godtfredsen J, Andersen ED & Andersen B (1989). Placebo-controlled, randomized trial of warfarin and aspirin for prevention of thromboembolic complications in chronic atrial fibrillation: the Copenhagen AFASAK Study. *Lancet* **1**, 175–9.

Pfeffer MA, Braunwald E, Moye LA *et al.*, on behalf of the SAVE Investigators (1991). Effect of captopril on mortality and morbidity in patients with left ventricular dysfunction after myocardial infarction. Results of the Survival and Ventricular Enlargement Trial. *N Engl J Med* **327**, 669–77.

PACK (Prevention of Atherosclerotic Complications with Ketanserin) Trial Group (1989). Prevention of atherosclerotic complications: controlled trial of ketanserin. *BMJ* **298**, 424–30.

RITA-2 (Second Randomised Intervention Treatment of Angina) Trial Participants (1976). Coronary angioplasty versus medical therapy for angina: the second Randomised Intervention Treatment of Angina (RITA-2) trial. *Lancet* **350**, 461–68.

RITA Trial Participants (1993). Coronary angioplasty versus coronary artery bypass surgery: the Randomised Intervention Treatment of Angina (RITA) Trial. *Lancet* **341**, 573–80.

Sacks FM, Pfeffer MA, Moye LA, Rouleau JL, Rutherford JD, Cole TG, Brown, Warnica JW, Arnold JMO, Wun CC, Davis BR & Braunwald E (1996). The effect of pravastatin on coronary events after myocardial infarction in patients with average cholesterol levels. *N Engl J Med* **335**, 1001–9.

Scandinavian Simvastatin Survival Study Group (1994). Randomised trial of cholesterol lowering in 4,444 patients with coronary heart disease: the Scandinavian Simvastatin Survival Study (4S). *Lancet* **344**,1383–9.

Schwartz PJ, Camm AJ, Frangin G, Janse MJ, Julian DG & Simon P, on behalf of the EMIAT Investigators (1994). Does amiodarone reduce sudden death and cardiac mortality after myocardial infarction? *Eur Heart J* **15**, 620–4.

Shepherd J, Cobbe SM, Ford I, Isles CG, Lorimer AR, Macfarlane PW, McKillop H& Packard CJ (1995). Prevention of coronary heart disease with pravastatin in men with hypercholesterolaemia. *N Engl J Med* **333**, 1301–7.

SOLVD Investigators (1992). Effect of enalapril on mortality and the development of heart failure in asymptomatic patients with reduced left ventricular ejection fractions. *N Engl J Med* **327**, 685–91.

Stroke Prevention in Atrial Fibrillation Investigators (1994). Warfarin versus aspirin for prevention of thromboembolism in atrial fibrillation. Stroke Prevention in Atrial Fibrillation II Study. *Lancet* **343**, 687–91.

Swedberg K, Held P, Kjekshus J, Rasmussen K, Ryden L & Wedel H, on behalf of the CONSENSUS II Study Group (1992). Effects on the early administration of enalapril on mortality in patients with acute myocardial infarction. Results of the cooperative new Scandinavian enalapril survival study II (CONSENSUS II). *New Engl J Med* **327**, 678–84.

Veterans Affairs Stroke Prevention in Nonrheumatic Atrial Fibrillation Investigations (1992). Warfarin in the prevention of stroke associated with nonrheumatic atrial fibrillation. *N Engl J Med* **47**, 06–2.

Waldo AL, Camm AJ, de Ruyter H *et al.*, for the SWORD Investigators (1996). Effect of d-sotalol on mortality in patients with left ventricular dysfunction after recent and remote myocardial infarction. *Lancet* **348,** 7–12.

Wilcox RG, Hampton JR, Banks DC *et al.* (1986) Trial of early nifedipine in acute myocardial infarction: the TRENT Study. *BMJ* **293**,1204–8.

Wilcox RG, Von der Lippe G, Olsson CG, Jensen G, Skene AM & Hampton JR, for The Anglo-Scandinavian Study of Early Thrombolysis Group (1990). Effects of alteplase in acute myocardial infarction: 6-month results from the ASSET Study. *Lancet* **335**, 1175–8.

Chapter 6

Evidence, guidelines, audit and oncology: principles and problems in primary, secondary and tertiary care

Roger D James, Michael Vaile, Anita Burrell, Daniel Jackson and Alan Alderson

Introduction

The National Institute for Clinical Excellence (NICE) will provide national service frameworks (guidelines/algorithms/protocols) which will be audited by the Commission for Health Improvement (CHI) according to a series of agreed parameters (minimum datasets) (NHS Executive 1999a). The chairman of NICE, Professor Sir Michael Rawlins, is a clinical pharmacologist. The chairman of CHI, Dame Deirdre Hine, was co-author of the Calman-Hine Report (Expert Advisory Group on Cancer 1995), which effectively set the standard and principle for altering the configuration of cancer services in the National Health Service (NHS). National service frameworks published so far for mental health and coronary heart disease are brief and the machinery for involving doctors and allied professionals in their implementation is yet to be made clear. The draft service framework for cancer (NHS Executive 1999b) contains recommendations on the constitution of the cancer management team: lead clinician, nurse, manager; network management; referral; education and training; diagnostic, radiotherapy, chemotherapy services.

The NICE-CHI auditing process will result in a framework of 'clinical governance issues', which will encourage 'self-regulation' and 'lifelong learning' (Miles *et al.* 2000). NICE will have the job of evaluating the most 'cost-effective' approach to a series of conditions, particularly in the secondary and tertiary (hospital-based) sectors. Recent NICE reviews have defined categories of licensed drug indications which the NHS will or will not reimburse. Cancer provides an ideal way of assessing the usefulness of this process, since multiple conditions are unusual, particularly in younger patients, and survival times are well documented. Cancer in the UK is characterised by low survival rates and low proportional per-capita expenditure compared with the rest of Western Europe. However, data on cancer registration and quality assurance (QA) around the delivery of cancer care in the UK are robust compared with those in other countries.

Recent changes in NHS administrative and advisory structure

The Thatcher administration introduced NHS reforms based on a split between purchaser and provider with devolution of fiscal and, to some extent, disciplinary responsibility to trust level. The Blair administration removed some fiscal independence from general practitioners (GPs) but introduced the idea of GP commissioning of secondary services. NICE and CHI are regulatory bodies whose activity will clearly affect primary (GP), secondary (cancer unit) and tertiary (cancer centre) cancer care provision. Government initiatives during 1999 like the Cancer Collaborative (National Patient's Access Team 1999) and the appointment of the 'Cancer Czar' suggest the need for a 'fast-track' advisory and delivery structure which may not conform to traditional NHS patterns.

The Calman-Hine report suggested that services for less common cancers such as leukaemia, gynaecological or head and neck cancers should be based on a population rather than a hospital. The report also recommended, based on published evidence, a multidisciplinary team approach to cancer site-specialisation involving a surgeon, oncologist, pathologist, radiologist and nurse. Inevitably, such a change alters the traditional referral pattern of suspected cancer patients from individual GPs to individual consultant surgeons or physicians. Recent NHS Executive communications suggest that primary and secondary sectors are now expected to collaborate around a common referral machinery for cancer patients that may not stipulate a certain named consultant. Over the last four years a series of managed care pathways (guidelines) and minimum datasets have been published by a variety of bodies, including the Royal Colleges and the NHS Executive. Increasingly, cancer services will be organised into networks, with a need to review the machinery of management and clinical governance. Essential policy features of a cancer network include evidence-based, patient-centred guidelines, a national service framework, re-engineering of the process of care delivery and real-time data collection.

In the UK clinical governance remains a chief executive responsibility in hospitals but will be introduced to the primary sector through primary care groups (PCGs) and trusts (PCTs). The General Medical Council (GMC) has added revalidation to its regulatory powers (Buckley 1999) but the profession has conceded that the NHS Executive should use CHI to deal with poor clinical performance (British Medical Association News Review 1999).

Antecedents of NICE and CHI

Quality assurance (QA)

There is an urgent need to regulate the service delivery of cancer surgery, radiotherapy and chemotherapy in the UK. Regional variations in cancer waiting times, mastectomy rates, the use of cytotoxic drugs and cancer cure rates are now deemed unacceptable. There is a public perception that the needs of patients are not addressed by health professionals. At the same time patients with cancer should have rapid access to diagnosis and treatment, with no waiting lists and investigations or treatments arranged around a work- or domestic schedule. Family and friends should have access to patients and their professional carers. Emergencies should be dealt with promptly and clinical research encouraged. However, the hospital sector of the NHS has witnessed a number of serious incidents over the last five years. In addition to the Bristol paediatric cardiac surgery case, there have been failures in cervical cancer screening and radiotherapy accidents in Exeter and Stoke. Each inquiry has led to a rise in litigation, public criticism of regulatory procedures and recommendations that QA systems become more accurate and reflexive than their predecessors.

QA data have been collected by the NHS for several years. These include those for notifiable diseases, cancer registries and confidential enquiries, such as those into perinatal and maternal mortality. However, the machinery for this sort of data collection is retrospective and responds poorly to innovation or adverse events. QA issues around clinical expertise remain partly the responsibility of health employers such as trusts (clinical governance), partly of the GMC (registration and revalidation) and partly of the Royal Colleges (CME programmes). QA can follow a number of models, but its strategic aim, achieved against a standard such as a manual or protocol, is to prevent rather than respond to failure. Clinical involvement in QA in the cancer field includes the QA of radiotherapy departments, the breast or cervical screening programme and clinical trials.

QA in radiotherapy

Radiotherapy departments in the UK are structurally regulated around the quality of equipment and staffing. Radiotherapy process QA monitors procedures such as machine calibration and staff protection. The definition of the term 'quality' is not generally well understood (Miles *et al.* 1995). It is commonly taken to intimate a degree of excellence. British Standard BS 4778 defines quality as 'the totality of features and characteristics of a product or service that bear upon its ability to satisfy stated or implied needs'. When defined in this way, it is clear that the assurance of quality depends upon the effective management of all the processes within an organisation that influence the satisfaction of customer need. In this context, 'customers' are first and foremost the radiotherapy patients of the oncology department, but also the oncologists and radiographers who use the oncology equipment, quality-assured by the medical physics department. The physics department's structure, responsibilities, resources, procedures and protocols necessary to satisfy its customers' needs and expectations are collectively called its 'quality system'. The quality system enables effective quality management to be implemented to maintain proper control of the whole process. The establishment of a system of quality management based on ISO 9000 is fundamental to accruing the full benefits of a quality assurance programme and should further lead to adopting the desirable practice of 'total quality management', the ultimate development of quality systems.

Quality Assurance in Radiotherapy (the 'QART' document) was the report of a working party under the chairmanship of Professor Norman Bleehen published in May 1991 (DoH 1991). The working party examined the whole issue of quality management in radiotherapy departments and made recommendations for the implementation of a documented quality system into radiotherapy practice, setting out 18 requirements to be satisfied. The ISO 9000 quality system applied to oncology was trialled at the Christie Hospital, Manchester, and at the Bristol Oncology Centre, using two different models. 'QART' introduced a seed change into 'quality' thinking within radiotherapy and this has begun to spread to other NHS services.

Practical quality assurance for radiotherapy has developed in two ways as a direct result of 'QART'. First, there is a UK initiative for dosimetry intercomparison that has evolved into a national audit programme. Eight audit groups have been set up covering the whole country. Each group contains a number of hospitals (NHS and private) which provide radiotherapy services. Each hospital's physics department audits another within their group in either a 'spoke' or 'circular' model, the model varying slightly between the eight groups. There is a single link between all eight groups, which also includes the UK's prime calibration dosimetry standard laboratory, the National Physical Laboratory (NPL), Teddington.

The audit includes both procedural and dosimetric aspects. Thus local QA procedures in use and application of dosimetry codes of practice are audited. There are dosimetric codes of practice for kilovoltage X-rays, megavoltage photon beams and electrons published by the Institute of Physics and Engineering in Medicine (IPEM) used throughout the UK, which are in line with internationally recognised standards of dosimetry. Additionally, one hospital's definitive dose calibration is checked by another using the other's own electrometer and ionisation chamber combination with its own separately derived calibration factors traceable to NPL, to independently verify that calibration. The calibration phantom used is based upon the IPEM-designed trapezoid phantom used for the first national dose intercomparison carried out in 64 radiotherapy centres (62 NHS + 2 private) between 1987 and 1991. There is a proposal to move toward an Edinburgh-designed semianatomical phantom, which will aid a more realistic assessment of that part of the dose audit usually carried out which checks a sample treatment plan, so including the performance of the therapy planning system in use. An independent audit is always carried out prior to the introduction of a new modality into clinical service in any UK radiotherapy department.

A variety of quality assurance tests are carried out routinely on radiotherapy equipment. These tests have evolved through individual UK hospitals developing their own QA protocols and standards over the years, coming to a consensus view on the important parameters and their required precision, accuracy and reproducibility, leading to the publication of *Physics Aspects of Quality Control in Radiotherapy* (IPEM 1999). The report states that quality assurance programmes must be structured to meet the clinical requirements for accuracy necessary to achieve optimum treatment outcome in terms of maximising tumour control probability and minimising normal tissue complications. It gives advice for setting up a quality assurance management programme to achieve this objective by defining the important parameters to check, their allowable tolerances and the ideal frequency of performing the check measurements.

The UK quality control protocol presented in IPEM Report 81 examines quality assurance and its conceptual framework within the radiotherapy context. Systematic approaches to quality assurance and audit are considered in terms of the 'QART' recommendations and the international quality standard ISO 9000. The complete radiotherapy process, including imaging, treatment planning, treatment machines and dosimetry for external beam treatments and for brachytherapy are covered in these national recommendations for QA. Recommendations are also made for quality assurance in *in-vivo* dosimetry and portal image verification.

Screening programmes, clinical trials

Breast- and cervical-screening programmes monitor the proportion of patients recalled because of inadequate samples and utilise random external review of smears or mammograms, which are proxy measures of outcome. The specificity and sensitivity of a screening programme determine its cost-effectiveness and feasibility. The incidence of cervical cancer, but not breast cancer, is falling in the UK and this is attributed to a costly screening programme. Cancer network initiatives like rapid-access, 'one-stop' clinics can be assessed for feasibility using screening QA methodologies. Drug registration and licensing bodies dealing with novel cytotoxic drugs demand clinical trials with high-level QA. These expensive exercises are usually commercially sponsored. They include strict structural QA around the enrolment of suitable centres and clinicians, process monitoring of compliance with protocol requirements on drug delivery, dose reductions and dose delays. A series of outcome measures include externally reviewed response, quality of life and toxicity data probably best achieved using clinical trial methodology.

In prospective clinical trials a group of stakeholders produce a protocol. Stakeholders include scientists, funding bodies, clinicians, health economists and psychologists. The protocol defines at the outset a novel therapeutic intervention, a population, an outcome measure and a statistical methodology. Data are collected prospectively and jointly owned. The trial funding body will often set up an independent monitoring committee and withdraw support if recruitment is inadequate. Most prospective clinical trials collect data for a specific purpose: in order to measure the impact of an innovation on a few, specific outcome measures. This investigation of cause and effect is not a primary aim of methodological audit, which is a form of process QA. Clinical trials are more likely than audit to produce a consensus protocol, define a patient population and statistical methodology in advance and correct for case-mix bias.

International trends

The UK, like most westernised societies, faces a fiscal crisis in health and welfare provision for an increasingly aged, retired population. As new interventions emerge and/or patients live longer with chronic conditions such as cancer, health-funding agencies are exposed to a liability risk. Many of the ideas behind the NHS reforms of the Thatcher administration were derived from insurance-funded health schemes. The exposure of third-party insurers in the USA to commercial risk has led to the practice of collaborative managed care. A sound, actuarial interpretation of published evidence very similar to that proposed for NICE is essential for risk-management. The cost of treating an individual with, say, lung cancer is part of an insurance risk similar to the cost-benefit assessment proposed by NICE. The introduction of 'collaboratives' between insurance funders and hospital providers is a US response to an increasingly competitive market. QA in such collaboratives is clearly a commercial issue. Doctors are unlikely to be employed by collaboratives unless they can show they are recertified on a regular basis by professional bodies. Assessment of clinical performance by patients forms an important part of collaborative programmes.

Concerns about NICE from the medical profession and pharmaceutical industry

Advisory machinery

Although some cancer initiatives like breast and cervical screening have been successful, many others, such as the two-week waiting-time target for cancer patients, are not evidence-based. Blocks to patient flow are generated by excess of demand over capacity and the site of such blocks in different trusts could include staff shortages in diagnostic radiology, pathology or secretarial services. Trust mergers and capital programmes can delay the installation of equipment like linear accelerators. Professional groups should therefore have input into the implementation process of policy initiatives, perhaps at regional level, perhaps through regional advisory committees. The cancer networks needed to deliver policies like screening and waiting-time reduction should be adequately costed, staffed and resourced using professional advice (Berwick *et al.* 1998).

Professional regulation and revalidation

Regulatory bodies should themselves be morally and intellectually accountable if they recommend unachievable standards. If the current advisory machinery for NICE or for the 'Cancer Czar' proves inadequate, it deserves reforming. Health authorities and trust managers need clear advice regarding the standards they should expect for clinical governance and audit. In Calman-Hine multidisciplinary teams, it may not be clear who holds clinical governance responsibility for individual patients. Regulation and revalidation are clearly related and their delivery will require professional consultation.

Patients with cancer move in and out of the voluntary (hospice) or private sectors. The central regulatory machinery of CHI should therefore be adapted for these realities and for the Calman-Hine concept of flexible, collaborative cancer networks. National service frameworks remain somewhat rarified statements of principles and standards and will be difficult to monitor for regulation without local interpretation and implementation. Guidelines exclude costs/toxicity of treatment and rapidly become out of date. Cost-effectiveness is less easy to define in general medicine than in surgery or service specialties such as radiology and pathology. Multiple conditions are common in the elderly population that frequents NHS hospitals. Transferring radiotherapy, screening or commercial drug trial QA into other areas of the NHS is likely to be complex and expensive. MRC (1998) advice on good clinical practice in clinical trials is less rigorous than similar pharmaceutical publications. There is a danger that guidelines will be used as a 'recipe' or 'map' for individual patients in direct contradiction of a policy of patient-centred care. They may respond sluggishly to strategic innovations and obscure glaring impediments to patient access such as staff shortages.

Data collection

It is difficult at this stage to see how NICE will separate its financial concerns for the NHS from an independent assessment of the science of innovation. The provision of the evidence for NICE to consider will itself cost money. Evidence independent of commercial interests can only be derived from sources like the MRC. The research infrastructure of the NHS needs to be maintained and expanded to provide relevant data. The national service framework for cancer will need to define process and outcome measures in order for NICE to monitor QA. The most accurate way of collecting unbiased outcome data is by using clinical trial methodology in which statistical power is defined prior to uniform data collection. Whoever funds and collects this 'new' type of evidence controls the coinage of health improvement. It is well known that the design and methodology of data collection determine outcome (Nelson *et al*. 1998). The medical profession has cast doubt on the usefulness of much of the retrospective NHS data collection used for cancer registries and audit programmes. These are perceived as being uncorrected for case variables, systematically biased and unable to manage rapid innovation. It is imperative that the quality of evidence collected conforms with that required from international, peer-reviewed journals. The professions should be involved in a debate with NICE over acceptable comparators and endpoints.

Concerns from the pharmaceutical Industry

The Association of the British Pharmaceutical Industry (ABPI 1999) has noted that 'NICE is an opportunity'. ABPI feels that 'it is important that guidance for NICE, as well as assessing clinical and cost effectiveness, should encourage innovation and be based on an integrated and holistic view of healthcare delivery. Its criteria should be transparent, reflecting a clear recognition of patient needs and support the twin aims of quality and equity in the NHS'.

The role of NICE is to appraise interventions before and after they are introduced into the NHS. This may have major implications for medicine development in Britain, and the availability of medicines to the NHS. Improving standards of patient care is a major challenge, and obviously will not be attained purely by the appraisal of pharmaceutical products. The development of clear, concise and timely guidelines is the ultimate goal of NICE, hopefully bringing to an end the problem of so called 'postcode prescribing'.

NICE will appraise health technologies, be they devices, pharmaceuticals or other, where it is considered that there is an inequitable distribution, or confusion about the most appropriate treatment to use. NICE guidelines should ensure a consistent approach to the adoption of new technologies to the potential benefit of all patients in the UK. NICE wishes to adhere to the principles of evidence-based medicine, which involves appraising all the evidence available for the intervention in a methodical, explicit and repeatable way. If the same methodology is applied to all the interventions appraised by NICE, then NICE guidance should be the common yardstick for health care interventions.

There are a number of concerns that are specific to the pharmaceutical industry, associated with NICE. The new evidence that has to be gathered to meet the needs of this body could dramatically add to the development costs of any pharmaceutical product. The trials currently undertaken are designed to illustrate the efficacy, safety and quality of the product. This means that they are only a specific indicator of the cost-effectiveness of the intervention in the UK marketplace. These trials are designed to examine pre-chosen *scientific* endpoints. Therefore the trial population is not entirely representative of the UK population as a whole. The *economic* data that can be attained from these trials as they stand are therefore limited to represent this specific population. The true cost-effectiveness of products can only be assessed once a specific product is in widespread use. NICE assessments therefore need to be a dynamic process evaluating the product in general practice as well as randomised controlled studies. Indeed, the ABPI has suggested that the product should be appraised fully only 'after an agreed period of general use'.

There are potential impacts on the development and introduction of medical interventions in the UK. If it is far more expensive to develop the product in the UK due to the different nature of the evidence required, then there is an incentive to move the development to other European countries without such requirements. This could affect the current high standing of the UK research base. A progression of this argument is that new products could cease to be launched in the UK. Another European country may offer a less problematic launch, and create the potential for further data to be collected, at less cost, before a UK launch is considered. This would run counter to the idea of reducing inequities in access to innovative treatments, as their availability in the UK would be delayed.

The UK has an innovative and highly competitive pharmaceutical industry, bringing significant benefits to the economy, the NHS and to patients. Constructive evolution of NICE in a way that does not inhibit innovation will be an important factor in the future of the UK-based pharmaceutical industry. NICE has undertaken a transparent and dynamic development process, actively consulting with the pharmaceutical industry. This process may resolve the concerns expressed above. It is a difficult road but there is a great need for dialogue so that all parties concerned can work towards the common goal of improved patient care.

Recommendations

Managed cancer care and managed cancer networks

The modern NHS is faced with the problem of ever-increasing demand on resources from a fast-growing ageing population, and the issue of making the best treatment choices, with regard to value for money when faced with an increasing number of treatment options. This dilemma inevitably leads to rationing of one form or another. What is required is a rationing method which can be seen to be fair with the patient at the centre of health care delivery.

Most cancer networks deliver a proportion of patients for tertiary care to the cancer centre and concern a population of between one and two million. Health authority and trust mergers would probably result in a network of one cancer centre with one health authority, three hospital trusts and four to five PCGs. Each cancer network is a 'virtual service organisation' and will need a management or policy board which pulls together all stakeholders, including patient groups, and an efficient policy of data transfer. Process QA in health management is increasingly dominated by electronic data transfer similar to that used by industry, such as commercial electronic expert a corporate website and a confidential real-time internal network.

Monitoring the process of care delivery in cancer

Policies generated by the network cancer policy board are based on national service frameworks and adopted, after consultation, by all stakeholders as clinical governance and QA protocols. A QA protocol is the essential language of a network. Cancer protocols are generally called 'guidelines', but are used to define the patient-pathway within the cancer network. As patients move, they fulfil the entry requirements for the next stop on the protocol. For example, a patient will only be booked into a one-stop breast clinic if the GP can satisfy national guidance on access (the patient has been examined, has a breast lump and is of the age to suggest it may be malignant). If these criteria, on assessment, are inefficient, resulting in an excess of non-malignant conditions, they should be modified. In this way, a continual feedback loop renders the processes controlled by a protocol more explicit, precise and up to date. A national service specification for cancer should be turned into a local cancer network protocol and monitored during its delivery. Guidelines can only be tested by using them.

Setting up local machinery for the QA of process and outcome encourages stakeholding, consensus and research and should be based on advice from a multidisciplinary 'disease-oriented group' (DOG). Each DOG for each of the common cancers comprises stakeholders from patient focus groups, funding/management bodies (health authority and trust chief executives and cancer lead clinicians) and provider units (PCHTs, surgeons, oncologists, nurses, radiologists, pathologists). Oncologists, GPs and experienced patients provide site-specialised, multidisciplinary teams. Health authority and trust chief executives provide the machinery for commissioning, funding, clinical governance and accreditation.

To show that change has occurred, QA should be linked to the process and outcome of the cancer network as well as to its structure. Each DOG has the same terms of reference each financial year, and it is accredited under clinical governance according to the delivery of three related processes. These are: (a) a protocol or patient-pathway for specific types of cancer, derived from national guidelines; (b) a minimum data-set for specific types of cancer and specific points on the patient pathway, collected using electronic data transfer – the responsibility for delivering these data rests with providers; and (c) a policy for integrating into clinical governance the prospective monitoring of the quality of patient care and modification of the protocol – the responsibility for clinical governance rests with health authority/trust nominees.

References

[ABPI] Association of The British Pharmaceutical Industry (1999). *NICE and medicines.* Leaflet BSC 6/99/4K.

Berwick D & Nolan T (1998). Physicians as leaders in improving health care. *Annals of Internal Medicine* **128**, 289–92.

British Medical Association News Review (1999). November, 18–24.

Buckley G (1999). Revalidation is the answer. *BMJ* **319**, 1145–6.

Department of Health (1991). *Quality assurance in radiotherapy. Report of a working party.* Chairman Professor Norman Bleehen. DoH, London.

Expert Advisory Group on Cancer (1995). *A policy framework for commissioning cancer services.* DoH, London.

[IPEM] Institute of Physics and Engineering in Medicine (1999). *Physics aspects of quality control in radiotherapy.* IPEM, York.

Miles A, Bentley P, Polychronis A & Grey J (1995). Purchasing quality in clinical practice: what on Earth do we mean. *Journal of Evaluation in Clinical Practice* **1**, 87–95.

Miles A, Hill A & Hurwitz B (eds.) (2000). *Clinical governance: enabling excellence or imposing control?* Aesculapius Medical Press, London (in press).

[MRC] Medical Research Council (1998). *MRC guidelines for good clinical practice in clinical trials.* MRC, London.

National Patient's Access Team (1999). *Cancer services collaborative handbook.* NPAT, Leicester.

Nelson E, Splaine M *et al.* (1998). Building measurement and data collection into medical practice. *Annals of Internal Medicine* **128**, 460–6.

NHS Executive (1999a). *Faster access to modern treatment: how NICE appraisal will work.* NHSE, Leeds.

NHS Executive (1999b). *National core standards for cancer services.* NHSE, Leeds.

Chapter 7

The selective use by NHS management of NICE-promulgated guidelines: a new and effective tool for systematic rationing of new therapies?

Stephen Harrison and George Dowswell

Introduction

The title of this chapter is full of loaded terms. Klein *et al.* (1996) have observed that, despite its etymology, the term 'rationing' prompts unreason. From the perspective of many practising physicians, 'management' is still a dirty word unless applied to diseases or patients. Even 'systematic' (which would be a term of approbation when used to describe a literature review) acquires sinister overtones in this context. Yet there is almost certainly a significant medical constituency which would not only answer 'yes' to the question in the title, but would take such an answer to be a sweeping condemnation of the National Institute for Clinical Excellence (NICE), the Commission for Health Improvement (CHI) and clinical governance. But the use of rhetoric is not the sole preserve of critics of the newest set of NHS reforms; the very titles of these new institutions exude goodness and reassurance, and even the jocular usage of 'CHIMP' rather than 'CHI' is discouraged.

So the question in our title is worth addressing, in the hope that we may be able to get behind some of the rhetoric. This is not, of course, to suggest that the rhetoric is unimportant; to the extent that it shapes actors' perceptions of situations, rhetoric can be a decisive political factor. Our exploration of the question is structured as follows. First, we seek to establish that rationing, in the sense that not everyone can have all their demands met, is inevitable in a system of third-party payment for health care like the NHS. The questions which those responsible for such systems must address, either explicitly or implicitly, are: who should make rationing decisions, according to what implicit or explicit criteria, and by what mechanisms should these decisions be implemented? Second, we note New Labour's answers to these questions. In the third section, we ask whether these are *defensible* answers. Finally, we ask how far they are likely to be *effective* answers.

Rationing health care

The principle of 'third-party payment' underpins not just the UK National Health Service (NHS) and other tax-financed health care systems, but also systems financed through social or private insurance. The principle is that financial contributions are collected from population groups, irrespective of the immediate health care requirements of the individuals who compose them. These contributions are collected by 'third-party payers', such as government or quasi-independent agencies or insurance companies, who employ the resources thus obtained to resource or reimburse health care providers for the care of individuals. Such systems can therefore be seen as pooling resources to avoid the possibility that individuals' health states may require more expenditure than the individual is able to afford. Unlike out-of-pocket payment, third-party payment does not limit the value of care provided to an individual to the sum of his or her contributions. Unfortunately, such arrangements risk the inflation of demand over time. While this is often conceptualised as being 'driven' by variables such as ageing populations, technological drift, and/or rising public expectations, they are not sufficient conditions. Demand increases are more appropriately theorised in terms of two tendencies derived from the economic concept of 'moral hazard': supplier-induced demand and consumer moral hazard (Arrow 1963).

Supplier-induced demand arises from information asymmetries; the consumer's lack of knowledge of a highly technical service coincides with a provider's interest in increasing provision and allows the latter to affect demand. Although patients do make generalised demands in the sense of arranging a visit to the doctor or being taken to the Accident Department, it is typically (though not invariably) the physician who translates this into a specific demand for a specific investigation or intervention. The professional motivation may be material; if the clinician is remunerated on a fee-for-service basis, there are incentives to maximise supplier-induced demand unless the total fees are 'capped' in some way, and the same incentive may exist if the institution which employs the clinician is itself remunerated by the third-party payer, either on the basis of its actual costs or on any basis which is volume-sensitive. If this were a complete explanation of motivation, an NHS in which clinicians are salaried or capitated would have the opposite effect, since there would be no incentives to perform beyond the level necessary to retain one's job. However, consideration only of material incentives seems unrealistically narrow. There may be ethical incentives for supplier-induced demand; even if the hospital's budget is not volume-related and clinicians are remunerated by salary, one might still expect to see such demand increase as a result of the supplier's desire to behave ethically, that is to do the best possible for his or her patient.

Consumer moral hazard arises because some or all of the costs of care are met by the third-party payers; it encourages a higher rate of use than would occur if full costs had to be met at the point of use (Pauly 1968), since the demander assumes that the cost of his or her usage will not relate directly to his or her present or future contributions. Third-party payment makes it easier for many people to obtain care than would otherwise be the case, but at the same time tempts them to increase their demands for services which they perceive as likely to be good for themselves. Such perceptions, which may or may not be justified, may be affected by media and Internet availability of information about health care (Coiera 1996) and the activity of patient pressure groups (Wood 2000). The diffusion of such information, along with the involvement of physicians in patient groups, blurs the distinction between supplier-induced demand and consumer moral hazard. However, the non-money costs of obtaining care can be significant. At the very minimum, the user must take steps, such as re-arranging a working day, travelling to the surgery or hospital, and perhaps waiting for some time, in order to gain access. Costs can be higher, for the treatment may be unpleasant, painful or even fatal.

Measures

Thus, demand in a third-party payment system might be expected to increase over time since neither consumers nor providers have the incentive to moderate it. This modern health care problem, of which the NHS is only one bearer, is a reflection of the way health care financing has been *collectivised* through the risk-pooling arrangements outlined above, and of how collectivisation, by breaking the direct link between consumption and payment, removes or weakens budget constraints on consumers. The responses available to a UK government can be roughly classified as follows (Harrison & Moran 2000). *Supply-side* measures aim to increase the flow of revenue to third-party payers (tax increases, charges, toleration of public sector budget deficits, and/or re-allocation of public expenditure priorities), or to encourage a higher level of out-of-pocket expenditure as an assumed substitute for third-party payment. Policy-makers may also seek to improve the productive efficiency of the sector by a range of management and organisational measures aimed at modifying the incentives facing providers. It is not necessary to imagine that demand is infinite in order to note that other countries choose to devote considerably greater resources to health care than does the UK without any apparent autonomous slackening of demand. Not surprisingly, few, if any, policy-makers or policy analysts believe that politically realistic supply-side measures alone are sufficient to meet rising demand, so that *demand-side* adjustments, aimed at reducing or containing demand for health care, have to be tolerated. Though the terminology is disputed, such adjustments are forms of 'rationing'.

Some such measures operate *implicitly* so far as the patient is concerned. Examples include the erection of cost barriers that partially offset the effect of consumer moral hazard. Such costs may be financial (thus charges for services are a deterrent), but spatial, psychological and procedural barriers may also be effective; remote or highly centralised facilities, user-unfriendliness, and strict 'gate-keeping' criteria tend to reduce demand. The doctrine of professional autonomy for clinicians has been an important safety valve, which has allowed rationing decisions to take place virtually invisibly (Aaron & Schwartz 1982; Harrison 1988). Other demand-side measures are *explicit*, that is consist of more-or-less clear rules about patient entitlement; for instance, such rules may exclude certain procedures or drugs.

Of course, these necessities are vigorously, if illogically, denied in official rhetoric. The arguments used in the White Paper, *The New NHS: Modern, Dependable*, to dismiss the need for rationing are largely fallacious; we can take three examples. First, it is stated that the Government rejects the need to ration, and asserts that 'so do the public'; this public rejection then turns out to be a normative preference for a universal service (Secretary of State for Health 1997, para 1.18). Second, it is argued that 'rising public expectations should be channelled into shaping services to make them more responsive to the needs and preferences of the people who use them' (ibid. para 1.19); it is hard to see how this is supposed to solve the problem, especially since an increase in the responsiveness of services seems likely to increase demand. Third, it is asserted that 'as technology advances [it allows] less invasive and hence cheaper treatments' (ibid., para 1.20); not only does this ignore the potential of less invasive treatments to be more acceptable to patients and thus *increase* demand, but it also ignores the fact that minimally invasive technology can be more expensive than traditional open surgical procedures. But it is clear that, whatever the terminology and rhetoric, UK governments are unable to eschew rationing. They must decide who is to ration, by what criteria and by what mechanisms (Harrison & Hunter 1994), either by condoning an arrangement by which it occurs (such as primary care gate-keeping or the use of clinical autonomy) or by actively intervening. The recent history of the NHS has been characterised by a slow shift from the former to the latter. The New Labour reforms embodied in clinical governance, national service frameworks, NICE and the guidelines which it will promulgate, and CHI represent the high point to date of this approach.

New Labour's answers

NICE was established in 1999 with three broad functions (NHS Executive 1998). First, it will make recommendations to the Government as to whether specific treatments are sufficiently cost-effective and affordable to be provided by the NHS. Second, it will give its imprimatur to 30–50 per annum 'evidence-based' clinical guidelines for the management of medical conditions. Third, it will be responsible for approving models of clinical audit for compulsory use by hospital doctors. In addition to this central specification of *clinical* models, there is to be central specification of *service* models, beginning with coronary heart disease and mental health. Thus 'national service frameworks' (NSFs) are being developed as a means of defining the pathway through primary, secondary and tertiary care which a particular type of patient will be expected to pass. CHI will be established as a statutory body and will 'conduct a rolling programme of reviews, visiting every ... Trust over a period of around 3–4 years' (ibid., pp.51–3). Such reviews will include local compliance with clinical guidelines issued by NICE, and with NSFs. In addition to routine reviews, the NHS management hierarchy will be able to initiate inquiries where local problems are suspected. Compliance with the products of these institutions will be a dimension of NHS performance management, providing a managerial motivation to respond (Black

1998). Chief executives will become responsible for the clinical, as well as the financial performance of their institutions and new legislation will place upon trusts a statutory duty for the quality of care. For each NICE guideline, a local 'lead clinician' will be identified as having responsibility for leading local implementation (NHS Executive 1998). The legal mechanisms by which the Government will enforce any decision that a treatment is insufficiently cost-effective for the NHS are not yet clear. It is, however, expected that NICE-approved clinical guidelines will normally be adhered to, and the chairman of NICE has publicly advised clinicians to record the reasons for any non-compliance in patient casenotes (Anon 1999a).

We can therefore discern New Labour's answers to the questions posed in the previous section. First, there will be greater involvement of the Government itself in rationing decisions, though it will be advised by NICE. Second, the chosen rationing criteria are largely explicit. Early official documents such as the 1997 White Paper focused on effectiveness as the underpinning principle for NICE, but more recent documents and comments from NICE's chairman have made it clear that matters of cost will also be considered (Anon 1999b), implying a shift to cost-effectiveness, perhaps a response to high-profile media treatment of expensive new interventions such as beta interferon and Viagra (sildenafil). Third, the aim of CHI and clinical governance is to provide a specific mechanism for rationing. Clinical governance is officially defined as:

> 'A framework through which NHS organisations are accountable for continuously improving the quality of their services and safeguarding high standards of care by creating an environment in which excellence in clinical care will flourish' (NHS Executive 1998, p.33).

This anodyne definition of clinical governance masks a significant challenge to clinical autonomy as previously practised; it amounts to the most systematic strategy for controlling doctors ever attempted in the NHS. In particular, NHS managers will, for the first time, have a strong incentive to seek to modify medical behaviour (see Miles *et al.* 2000).

Defensible answers?

Opponents of the New Labour reforms have their rhetoric too. We can examine two examples. First, the NHS reforms were not initially resisted by the medical profession; the manner of their reception was perhaps influenced by the media and public response to reports that paediatric cardiac surgeons in Bristol had a poor survival record for particular surgical procedures and that attempts by colleagues to draw attention to this had apparently been obstructed (Klein 1998). However, the BMA Annual Representatives Meeting of 1999 called on the organisation to monitor the activities of NICE and CHI 'to ensure that they [do] not develop into covert systems of rationing' (Anon 1999c). Yet we have seen that rationing is necessary and that New Labour's plans for it are more overt than covert. Second, 'Enabling excellence or imposing control?' is the subtitle of this volume. The juxtaposition of these phrases implies that they are antonyms, yet this is only partly the case. 'Enabling' and 'imposing' are indeed antonyms, but 'excellence' and 'control' belong to different conceptual orders and cannot therefore be antonyms. Put another way, there is no *necessary* contradiction between them and although the tact and diplomacy of policy-makers tend to leave them wary of seeming to 'impose' policies, blunter proponents of the reforms can argue that the means is irrelevant; it is undoubtedly defensible to argue that if excellence (that is, in this context, the implementation of cost-effective care) can be secured by imposing new controls on the medical profession, so be it.

Moreover, the criteria of effectiveness and cost-effectiveness are defensible definitions of 'excellence' though, as we shall see below, this does not mean that alternatives are not. The relative desirability of implicitness and explicitness is contentious (Mechanic 1992, 1997; Hoffenberg 1992; Hunter 1993; Harrison & Hunter 1994; Klein *et al.* 1996; New & Le Grand 1996). On the face of it, NICE's criteria will be explicit, a fact that ought to be welcomed or not, as the case may be, by commentators according to their prior position on the principle. (The present authors tend towards a preference for explicitness.) Moreover, the attractions of *clinical* effectiveness as a criterion for rationing are obvious. It can seem (or be made to seem) ludicrous to suggest that anyone might want ineffective care:

> *'Patients seek care in order to be relieved of some actual or perceived, present or potential, "dis-ease". The care itself is not directly of value; it is generally inconvenient, often painful or frightening. As a thought experiment, one could ask a representative patient (or oneself) whether he/she would prefer to have ... a condition perceived as requiring care plus the best conceivable care for that condition, completely free of all ... costs, or would prefer simply not to have the condition ... Care is not a good in the usual sense, but a "bad" or "regrettable" made "necessary" by the even more regrettable circumstances of "dis-ease". It follows that patients want to receive **effective** health care, i.e. care [in respect of which] there is a reasonable expectation [of] a positive impact on their health!'* (Evans 1990, pp.118–19, emphasis in original).

The defensibility of *cost*-effectiveness as a rationing criterion follows from two further considerations. First, given the rate of medical technical innovation and of public knowledge about it, there is every possibility that a single criterion of effectiveness would fail to rule out sufficient interventions to allow the NHS to operate within any conceivably realistic budget allocation. Cost-effectiveness would, in principle, allow a rank-ordering. Second, a criterion of cost-effectiveness helps to minimise opportunity costs – the possibility that substantial resources will be devoted to 'hopeless cases', while effective interventions are denied to patients with a substantial prospect of benefit. (It should be noted, however, that 'cost-effectiveness' in connection with NICE's role has been discussed in terms of 'affordability', which hardly corresponds to an economist's view of the concept: see, for instance, Anon (1999a), p.16.)

Finally, it seems likely that much of the emphasis of NICE's initial activity will continue to focus on new therapies. The pragmatic politics of such marginal analysis are understandable. It is precisely expensive new technologies such as those alluded to above that present themselves both as financial problems and as opportunities for action before they become embedded in routine practice with all the attendant ethical and political problems of withdrawal once established. Of course, such pragmatic politics could undermine the legitimacy of any claim to practise cost-effectiveness analysis since it leaves established clinical practices unquestioned.

If we are prepared to overlook misleading government rhetoric about rationing, NICE and the associated New Labour reforms can thus be seen as an honourable and defensible enterprise. Of course, it does not follow from this that the reforms are beyond criticism; to say that they are defensible does not mean that the case is 'watertight', only that it is not ridiculous. Alternative arguments as to how the problem of rationing is to be handled can and should be developed. Nor does it follow that the reforms will be effective. This is the subject of our final section.

An effective mechanism?

Despite their systematic nature and the energetic implementation arrangements outlined above, the probable effectiveness of the NICE/CHI reforms rests upon at least three assumptions, each of which looks commonsensical and yet is by no means unquestionable. In this section we question each of these: are rationing criteria of effectiveness and cost-effectiveness likely to command public and political support? Is the basis of 'evidence' from which NICE assessments are derived likely to be accepted by physicians and the public? Are the bureaucratic (a term used here in its technical sense) arrangements likely to modify medical behaviour in the desired fashion?

The acceptability of effectiveness and cost-effectiveness

The criteria of effectiveness and cost-effectiveness are not the only ones which surface in discussions about appropriate rationing criteria. One alternative is the *rule of rescue*, which gives priority to persons in acute or life-threatening conditions, and locates moral content in trying, rather than in succeeding. Although, as noted above, its application implies potentially significant opportunity costs, it is one which seems to receive wide support in public policy generally, underpinning as it does such services as air/sea rescue and mountain rescue. There is a cartoon in which a coastguard is answering a distress call with the words, 'Stay with your boat, Sir, whilst the Secretary of State decides how important you are'. It is far from obvious that such an outrageous suggestion would become any less outrageous by the substitution of, 'Stay with your boat, Madam, whilst the coastguard calculates whether the probability of getting to you in time is high enough to make it worth bothering'. Whatever its internal incoherence or unsought consequences, the rescue principle is one to which people subscribe. It is also the ostensible moral basis of medicine. Another alternative might be termed *entitlement*. Strictly speaking, UK citizens have few legal rights to publicly financed health care. Rather, the legalities are accomplished via the Secretary of State's statutory duty to provide a comprehensive health service. But this does not mean that people do not see themselves as having rights to treatment irrespective of calculations of effectiveness. Denied arterial surgery on the ground that his continued smoking increased the risks of treatment and reduced the probability of benefit, a 62-year-old Wakefield man was quoted as saying,

> *'I have worked since I was fourteen up until recently and paid a hell of a lot in taxes to the government both in income taxes and on the forty cigarettes a day I smoked. Surely it is not too much for me to ask to have an operation that might ease my pain in my old age and make me live a little longer'* (Anon 1993, p.1).

Of course, these examples are selected to illustrate our *a priori* point. Whatever the defensibility of effectiveness and cost-effectiveness as rationing criteria (as acknowledged above), it does not follow that public consensus is thereby obtained. Bluntly, other rationing criteria have their attractions too, and how the public and the media react to NICE is an empirical question which will no doubt be carefully monitored by policy-makers.

A related problem of acceptability is the lack of clarity as to how cost-effectiveness relates to *equity* of service distribution, since the ostensible rationale for third-party payment systems is to ameliorate the position of people who cannot afford the care from which they might benefit. New Labour's rather glib approach to this is to highlight 'postcode rationing' and geographical medical practice variations, interpreting equity as met by their abolition. It does not follow from this that everyone who has a need will have it met, a conclusion amply demonstrated in government decisions (later overturned by the courts) about the availability of the anti-impotence drug Viagra on aetiological, rather than diagnostic grounds (see Chapter 8).

Finally, even the single criterion of effectiveness is not straightforward in practice. It is not uncommon to find disputes about who is authorised to determine at what level of probability (or at what 'numbers-needed-to-treat') an intervention is counted as sufficiently effective for NHS provision. The notorious 'Child B' case illustrates this, but there have been others (Freemantle & Harrison 1993; New 1996). NICE seems to promise authoritative answers to such disputes, and to allow the rationing process to be defended with the authority of science. It is far from certain that the answers delivered will be seen as authoritative, for two reasons. First, there is ample evidence from public opinion polls that clinical doctors are the preferred agents of rationing, rather than politicians or managers. While it is certainly possible to argue that NICE's decisions are in some sense made by doctors, it does not follow that this is how matters will be seen by the public. Second, it is evident that the probability at which an intervention is counted as 'effective' is not medical or scientific (though it may be presented as such), but straightforwardly political; patient and user pressure groups are likely to be well aware of this.

The acceptability of evidence as defined by NICE

A second area about which the New Labour reforms make assumptions is the nature of the evidence which will underpin NICE's decisions. It has become a 'given' that evidence concerning the effectiveness of clinical interventions should be assessed in terms of its position in the so-called 'hierarchy of evidence', which privileges randomised controlled trials (RCTs) (Canadian Task Force 1979) and meta-analyses and systematic reviews of such trials. Not everyone, however, shares these assumptions; other epistemologies are defensible, and it does not follow that this approach is shared by rank-and-file physicians. The potential contrast is summarised in Table 7.1.

For the sake of contrast, Table 7.1 presents the two epistemologies as ideal types, though in the real world it seems likely that many clinicians are influenced by elements of both. The left-hand column represents the traditional model taught to clinicians. It treats the body as a kind of machine, relying on the discovery of cause-effect mechanisms by the observation of the way in which disease processes develop over time and impact upon normal physiological processes. Treatment is therefore very much a *logical* process of intervening in the aetiology (natural history) of a disease so as to arrest, reverse or retard it. Expressed in more philosophical/technical terms, the model is *deterministic* (that is, it assumes that clinical events necessarily have causes that can be identified and, in principle, modified). Learning in such a model is primarily from one's own experience. The right-hand column illustrates the conceptual underpinnings of the hierarchy of evidence. It consists primarily of the *inference* of cause-effect relationships from past statistical relationships between treatment and outcomes. It is therefore less concerned with disease processes than with establishing what interventions are *likely to be effective, irrespective of why*. The model is therefore *probabilistic* (that is, one where the cause-effect relationships are inherently uncertain) and relies on learning from an assembled body of scientific knowledge.

Table 7.1 Models of evidence in medicine

Traditional epistemology (working clinicians)	Scientific epistemology (outcomes researchers)
Reveals cause-effect mechanisms (via aetiology, pathology, etc); implied metaphor of the body as a machine	Demonstrates statistical relationships from past experience; implied metaphor of the body as a 'black box'
Provides knowledge of what logically ought to be effective, and why; 'logic of treatment' is important	Provides knowledge of what is *likely* to work, irrespective of why
Learning from experience	Learning from external sources
Based on deterministic models	Based on probabilistic models

Source: Adapted from Tanenbaum (1994)

The positions espoused by physicians have been the subject of a small-scale, but important US study (Tanenbaum 1994), which found that in the last analysis it was the traditional model that predominated in medical decision-making. A very practical consequence of these apparently rather abstruse observations is that clinical doctors are more likely to be influenced in their practice by their own (and close colleagues') experience with similar types of patient, and by their own reasoning about treatment logic, than by the publication of meta-analyses of large numbers of cases. In contrast, the health services research model places clinical observations at the bottom of the hierarchy of evidence. US physicians are not British physicians, and again it is a matter for empirical research to discover the epistemological positions espoused by the latter. It is worth noting, however, that the traditional position is highly consonant with the individualistic ethic of the practice of medicine and with the habit of doctors of being influenced by their own experience of particular cases. The regular 'filler boxes' in the *BMJ* with titles such as 'A memorable patient' may both reflect this habit and subvert the message of the RCTs reported in the adjacent columns (Harrison 1998).

Even if doctors were not hostile to the RCT model, an additional consideration is the view which they adopt about the generalisability of findings to their own patients as a group or as individuals. It is clear from the advice (cited above) that clinicians should record reasons for non-adherence to guidelines that such non-adherence is expected to be exceptional. Yet it is not clear whether clinicians themselves see matters in this way.

The effectiveness of the implementation model

The New Labour reforms assume that the essentially bureaucratic approach of NICE/CHI and clinical governance is most likely to impact on medical behaviour. We use the term 'bureaucracy' here in a technical sense; its defining features are instrumental (i.e. means-ends) rationality, specialisation, accountability, rules and hierarchy (Weber 1947). These elements are intended to provide efficiency, predictability and control, but it has long been evident that they may also have dysfunctions. Thus they may fail to utilise employees' intelligence, ignore the complex informal mechanisms found in every organisation and fail to adapt to external changes. Bureaucracies have also been seen to degenerate over time, with the following three processes recurring. First, rules accumulate but are not generally reviewed or repealed. This may lead to anachronistic or contradictory injunctions which undermine their credibility. Second, when mistakes occur, responsibility drifts upwards as a result of increasing managerial interest, hindering the possibility of learning and the exercise of discretion by those originally charged with carrying out the work. This disempowerment is unsustainable in the long term as practitioners become more alienated and managers more overloaded. Finally, 'goal displacement' may occur; the rules become 'sanctified' and attention focuses on adherence rather than the pursuit of wider or more appropriate aims (Heckscher 1994).

Unsurprisingly, awareness of increasingly rapid socio-technical change has caused research attention to be directed at the extent to which formal bureaucracies remain the most effective mechanism for management. Bureaucracy is traditionally considered to work best in environments which are relatively simple and stable, whereas conditions of complexity and more rapid change are perceived to require more 'organic', interactive or participative mechanisms (Heckscher & Applegate 1994), a finding which has been empirically identified in research in health services. Thus studies of the impact of quality improvement initiatives in US hospitals have suggested that organisational culture is likely to affect local uptake. Specifically, participative, flexible, risk-taking organisational culture was found to be strongly related to the implementation of quality improvement initiatives and better patient outcomes, whereas bureaucratic and hierarchical cultures were found to act as a barrier to implementation (Shortell *et al.* 1995). These considerations have also begun to enter analyses of clinical guideline implementation strategies in the UK. Thus Harrison (1994) has stressed the importance of organisational culture in this respect, and Grol (1992, 1997) has identified a spectrum of change strategies, from coercion and control to facilitation and education. Grol (1992) has criticised most guideline implementation strategies for narrowness and naïvety, pointing out that there is little evidence to support the use of coercive strategies and arguing that attention should be devoted to most parts of the implementation spectrum simultaneously. Studies of why UK medical practitioners change their clinical behaviour tend to support these arguments by indicating the multiple causal factors involved (Armstrong *et al.* 1996; Allery *et al.* 1997).

Concluding remarks

Let us summarise the argument of this chapter. First, rationing (as we have defined it) is a practical necessity for the NHS and probably has been throughout its existence. Rationing in accordance with one or more implicit or explicit criteria is unavoidable. Second, the aim of NICE, CHI and clinical governance is to provide a mechanism and specific criteria for rationing, probably concentrated in practice on new therapies. The criteria of effectiveness and cost-effectiveness are certainly defensible ones, though certainly not beyond argument or criticism. However, we have identified three sets of assumptions upon which the NICE/CHI and clinical governance reforms seem to be based, and pointed out that these may not be justified. First, it is not necessarily the case that there is a public and political consensus about the criteria of effectiveness and cost-effectiveness, and in any case the criterion of effectiveness is in practice as political as it is technical. Second, despite the apparent ascendancy of the view that 'good' evidence in respect of medical care interventions consists primarily of evidence drawn from RCTs, it does not follow either that most clinicians espouse this epistemology or that; if they do, they regard its conclusions as being more or less uniformly applicable to the patients in their care. Finally, the assumptions underpinning the implementation strategy for the reforms have to a large extent been superseded as a way of thinking about organisational change.

References

Aaron HJ & Schwartz WB (1984). *The painful prescription: rationing hospital care*. Brookings Institution, Washington (DC), USA.

Allery LA, Owen PA & Robling MR (1997). Why general practitioners and consultants change their clinical practice: a critical incident study. *BMJ* **314**, 870–4.

Anon (1993). *Yorkshire Evening Post*, 26 August.

Anon (1999a). NICE work. *BMA News Review*, March.

Anon (1999b). NICE to sort clinical 'wheat from chaff'. *BMJ* **318**, 416.

Anon (1999c). BMA Annual Representatives Meeting. *BMJ* **319**, 193.

Armstrong D, Reyburn H & Jones R (1996). A study of general practitioners' reasons for changing their prescribing behaviour. *BMJ* **312**, 949–52.

Arrow KJ (1963). Uncertainty and the welfare economics of medical care. *American Economic Review* **53**, 941–73.

Black N (1998). Clinical governance: fine words or action? *BMJ* **316**, 297–8.

Canadian Taskforce on the Periodic Health Examination (1979). Taskforce report: the Periodic Health Examination. *Canadian Medical Association Journal* **121**, 1139–254.

Coiera E (1996). The Internet's challenge to health care provision. *BMJ* **312**, 3–4.

Evans RG (1990). The dog in the night-time: medical practice variations and health policy. In *The challenge of medical practice variations* (ed. TF Andersen & G Mooney), Macmillan, Basingstoke.

Grol R (1992). Implementing guidelines in general practice care. *Quality in Health Care* **1**, 184–91.

Grol R (1997). Beliefs and evidence in changing clinical practice. *BMJ* **315**, 418–21.

Freemantle N & Harrison S (1993). Interleukin 2: the public and professional face of rationing in the NHS. *Critical Social Policy* **13**, 94–117.

Harrison S (1988). *Managing the National Health Service: shifting the frontier?* Chapman and Hall, London.

Harrison S (1994). Knowledge into practice: what's the problem? *Journal of Management in Medicine* **8**, 9–16.

Harrison S (1998). The politics of evidence-based medicine in the UK. *Policy and Politics* **26**, 15–32.

Harrison S & Hunter DJ (1994). *Rationing health care*. Institute for Public Policy Research, London.

Harrison S & Moran M (2000). Resources and rationing: managing supply and demand in health care. In *The handbook of social studies in health and medicine* (ed. G Albrecht, R Fitzpatrick & S Scrimshaw), pp.494–508. Sage, New York.

Heckscher C (1994). Defining the post-bureaucratic type. In *The post-bureaucratic organization: new perspectives on organizational change* (ed. C Heckscher & A Donnellon), pp.14–62. Sage, Thousand Oaks (CA), USA.

Heckscher C & Applegate LM (1994). Introduction. In *The post-bureaucratic organization: new perspectives on organizational change* (ed. C Heckscher & A Donnellon), pp.1–13. Sage, Thousand Oaks (CA), USA.

Hoffenberg R (1992). Letter to the editor. *BMJ* **304**, 182.

Hunter DJ (1993). Rationing and health gain. *Critical Public Health* **4**, 27–32.

Klein RE (1998). Competence, professional self-regulation and the public interest. *BMJ* **316**, 1740–2.

Klein RE, Day P & Redmayne S (1996). *Managing scarcity: priority setting and rationing in the National Health Service*. Open University Press, Buckingham.

Mechanic D (1992). Professional judgement and the rationing of medical care. *University of Pennsylvania Law Review* **140**, 1713–54.

Mechanic D (1997). Muddling through elegantly: finding the proper balance in rationing. *Health Affairs* **16**, 83–92.

Miles A, Hill A & Hurwitz B (eds.) (2000). *Clinical governance: enabling excellence or imposing control?* Aesculapius Medical Press, London (in press).

New B (1996). The rationing agenda in the NHS. *BMJ* **312**, 1593–601.

New B & Le Grand J (1996). *Rationing in the NHS: principles and pragmatism.* King's Fund, London.

NHS Executive (1998). *A first class service.* Department of Health, London.

Secretary of State for Health (1997). *The new NHS: modern, dependable.* Cm 3807. The Stationery Office, London.

Shortell SM, O'Brien JL, Carman JM, Foster RW, Hughes EFX, Boerstler H & O'Connor EJ (1995). Assessing the impact of continuous quality improvement/total quality management: concept versus implementation. *Health Services Research* **30**, 377–401.

Tanenbaum SJ (1994). Knowing and acting in medical practice: outcomes research. *Journal of Health Politics, Policy and Law* **19**, 27–44.

Weber M (1947). *The theory of social and economic organization.* Oxford University Press, New York, USA.

Wood B (2000). *Patient power? Patients' associations in Britain and America.* Open University Press, Buckingham.

Chapter 8

NICE and the ultimate decision makers: the legal framework for prescription and reimbursement of medicines

Ian Dodds-Smith

Introduction

This chapter seeks to explain the legal and historical context against which the National Institute for Clinical Excellence (NICE) will conduct its work but by reference to only one of the sectors affected by its constitution, namely the prescription and reimbursement of medicinal products under the National Health Service (NHS). NICE's remit, of course, goes further and covers devices, diagnostic techniques and other health issues but its creation owes much to the perceived inequities in the ability of patients to access new medicinal treatments and this field, therefore, illustrates well the Institute's powers and the limits to them.

The architecture of the NHS legislation

NHS legislation is complex and ever-changing but in the field of prescription reflects largely unchanged the original rationale for the Service. The 1944 White Paper, *A National Health Service,* had a clear vision:

> *'... to ensure in future every man and woman and child can rely on getting all the advice and treatment and care which they may need in matters of personal health; that what they get shall be the best medical and other facilities available; that their getting these shall not depend on whether they can pay for them, or on any other factor irrelevant to the real need'* (DoH 1944).

For successive governments, the test of their ability to be trusted with the NHS has appeared to be their willingness to stand by these principles. The essence of those principles was repeated in the *Patients' Charter* (DoH 1995a, p.5), which advises that patients have 'the right to ... receive healthcare on the basis of your clinical need, not on your ability to pay, your lifestyle or any other factor' (see also the European Social Chapter 1996, Article 13). The current Government came to power on a Manifesto (Anon 1997, p.20) that sought to allay fears that had surfaced from time to time with the previous Government, about whether that Government was encouraging a debate about the ability of the country to afford a NHS built on these principles:

'Labour commits itself anew to the historic principle: that if you are ill or injured there will be a national health service there to help; and access to it will be based on need and need alone – not on your ability to pay, or on who your GP happens to be or on where you live'.

Even today, the basic obligations of the Secretary of State under the National Health Service Act 1977 (the '1977 Act') are largely unchanged as compared with those imposed upon the first holder of that office. It is to promote a 'comprehensive' health service (Section 1 of the 1977 Act), which the 1944 White Paper stated meant first that it is available to all people and second that it covers all necessary forms of health care. But the Secretary of State's duty is also declared to be to provide medical services 'to such extent as he considers necessary to meet all reasonable requirements' (Section 3 of the 1977 Act). It must immediately be noted that these words import a significant amount of discretion. Not only does he have some latitude in determining what constitutes a 'reasonable requirement' but, as will be seen, the courts have accepted that in determining his obligations he must also have regard to the fact that public funds are not unlimited.

The Secretary of State arranges for the performance of his obligations through health authorities and special health authorities (and now through trust hospitals and primary care trusts). But the ultimate power rests with the Secretary of State – they are merely his agents delegated to perform functions under the 1977 Act. On his behalf, health authorities contract for the provision of general practitioners' services on the basis that they must ensure that patients receive 'adequate personal care and attendance' (Section 29 of the 1977 Act).

Advisory committees

To assist him in performing his functions the Secretary of State may constitute advisory committees as necessary and in the recent past we have seen one such committee (created pursuant to an Order made under Section 6 of the 1977 Act) – the Standing Medical Advisory Committee (SMAC) – play an increasing role in providing advice on how the NHS should take up new medicines. SMAC consists of members appointed by ministers from nominations made by the professions and includes the Presidents of the Royal Colleges. It has given advice on prescription of beta-interferons for multiple sclerosis in November 1995, statins in August 1997, Aricept (donepezil) in April 1998 and Viagra (sildenafil) in November 1998. In each case, however, it has tended to emphasise that its guidance does not supplant the fundamental right of the doctor to exercise his clinical judgement as he sees fit but is merely general guidance:

'... based upon the best evidence available at the moment on clinical effectiveness and long-term safety. It is not intended to replace or override clinical judgement in individual cases' (SMAC statement on use of statins, 1997).

NICE represents a further stage in the development of the advisory committee functions.

Prescription by general practitioners

The NHS legislation establishes the terms upon which general practitioners must be contracted to provide services in the area over which their health authority has control. These statutory terms of service are set out in Schedule 2 to the NHS (General Medical Services) Regulations 1992. They illustrate the aim of a comprehensive system by providing that each doctor should 'render to his patients all necessary and appropriate personal medical services of the type usually provided by general medical practitioners' (Schedule 2, para.12 of the 1992 Regulations). Doctors are invited to treat patients according to their clinical judgement in the light of the individual circumstances of each patient. There was originally no restriction on the products that could be prescribed – provided the product was given for a medicinal purpose. Reimbursement by the NHS would only be put in issue if the substance prescribed could not properly be described as a 'drug'. If a doctor prescribed what more properly should be treated as a cosmetic or food, he would have to justify its medicinal purpose to the relevant Local Medical Committee of the health authority (Regulation 36 of the 1992 Regulations)[1] and a failure to persuade that committee of the correctness of his stance might (subject to an appeal right to the Secretary of State) result in him having to meet the costs of the prescription himself.

Importantly, the over-arching principle that the NHS would meet all real clinical needs without need for the patient to have recourse to private treatment, led to the incorporation of anti-avoidance provisions as part of the statutory terms for general practitioners so as to stop private consultation or prescription. Once a clinical need was identified, the doctor was forbidden from charging a patient on his NHS list a fee for consultation and was forbidden from prescribing privately. To avoid circumvention, doctors in the same practice were forbidden from treating privately a patient referred to them by their partner.[2] This principle became controversial when prescription charges reached the point where a private prescription would, in some cases, be cheaper for the patient. It also led to particular difficulties when the Secretary of State sought in 1998 to stop the prescription of a new treatment for erectile dysfunction – Viagra (sildenafil) – on the NHS without black-listing the product using the appropriate legislative machinery.

Elucidation of the extent of the obligations of the Secretary of State

Successive decisions have shown that the English courts will intervene in the manner in which the Secretary of State performs his obligations only in limited circumstances.

---

1. Note, however, the proposals for wide clinical audit of GP performance and disciplinary action by health authorities contained in the Department of Health consultation document, *Supporting Doctors, Protecting Patients,* (November 1999), at Chapter 5.
2. Para.38 of the Terms of Service precludes a doctor (unless he is a dispensing doctor) from charging for treatment (including supply of the product) and paras 40 and 42 prohibit him and his partners from prescribing privately.

Shortly after cost pressures began to bite within the NHS, it was established that the Secretary of State's obligation to meet all reasonable requirements was subject to consideration of available resources. Having noted the pressures created on the NHS by both an ageing population and major scientific and technical advances in the treatment of all manner of ailments, Lord Denning *(R v Secretary of State for Social Services and others,* ex parte *Hincks* 1980) stated that it was a 'manifest illusion' that disappointed patients could appeal to the courts to enhance standards and ensure that their expectations were met:

> *'It cannot be supposed that the Secretary of State has to provide all the latest equipment ... [it] cannot be supposed that the Secretary of State has to provide all the kidney machines which are asked for, or all the new developments such as heart transplants in every case where people would benefit from them. It cannot be that the Secretary of State has a duty to provide everything that is asked for in the ... circumstances which have come about'.*

That is not to say that patients can expect no help from the courts where health authorities act irrationally, such as by seeking to exclude completely certain types of treatment using artificial distinctions as to what constitutes an illness for which a patient may have a legitimate expectation of treatment under the NHS. In July 1999 the decision by the Northwest Lancashire Health Authority to refuse any funding to transsexuals for sex change operations was declared illegal (*R v Northwest Lancashire Health Authority*, ex parte *G and others* 1999). The health authority in question had argued that, where there were limited funds available, it could effectively rule out the funding of such operations on the basis that they were not concerned with the treatment of illness but rather a state of mind which did not warrant medical treatment. The Court of Appeal, in upholding a decision against the health authority at first instance, noted that there is 'overwhelmingly evidence' that transsexualism is an illness that requires treatment. As will be seen in relation to the manner in which health authorities have acted upon NHS Circulars relating to the treatment of patients having multiple sclerosis with the new beta-interferons, the courts draw a distinction between prioritising treatment and, whether on cost grounds or otherwise, taking steps that, in practice, exclude it altogether.

The Court of Appeal noted that where an authority is obliged to make choices through lack of funds, it can take account of a wide range of considerations, including the proven success or otherwise of the proposed treatment, the seriousness of the condition to be treated and the cost of treatment. But any decision must be rationally based upon a proper consideration of the facts. The courts will look closely at the process by which decisions involving refusal of treatment in respect of a substantiated medical condition occur, especially if in practice they involve excluding the exercise of medical judgement on the individual circumstances of each case.

Influencing general practitioners as decision-makers

Despite the largely unfettered rights of doctors under the NHS legislation to determine the appropriate treatment for their patients, there has long been a history of providing advice to doctors that takes into account the cost of medicines. In the 1960s a Standing Joint Committee on the Classification of Proprietary Preparations (the Macgregor Committee) was established to provide advice to doctors about prescribing and to discourage the use of products of 'doubtful or unethical character' and those that were unnecessarily expensive (Anon 1965; see also Anon 1967). The Macgregor Committee operated before the Medicines Act 1968 was passed to create a system for the licensing of medicinal products based on an independent assessment of their safety, efficacy and quality. Products were divided into category A and category B preparations, with prescription of the latter requiring special justification if a doctor's prescribing were ever to be formally investigated. Having said that, the guidance noted that there remained 'no restriction upon a doctor prescribing any drug which, in his view, is necessary for the treatment of his patients ...'.

With the establishment of the Committee on the Safety of Drugs which metamorphosed into the Committee on Safety of Medicines in 1971 (when the licensing system under the 1968 Act became effective), part of the role of the Macgregor Committee disappeared and it became responsible only for advising on whether products should properly be treated as drugs at all. At that time it gained the new name of Advisory Committee on Borderline Substances (ACBS). The ACBS issues advice on products that should normally be treated as cosmetics, foods or disinfectants and initially that advice was not legally binding. It was made available to doctors in various ways, including through the British National Formulary, and if a doctor chose to ignore it, he could expect a difficult time justifying his actions when called to account by his health authority. From 1985, however, ACBS advice led to black-listing of products altogether.

The relevance of licensing

In the context of the creation of the licensing system, it should be noted that European medicines legislation, with which UK domestic legislation must be consistent, does not impinge upon the power of Member States to make their own decisions in relation to the pricing and reimbursement of medicinal products. The controlling legislation is Directive 65/65/EEC, which provides for the grant of a marketing authorisation when the applicant has established the quality, efficacy and safety of a product to the satisfaction of the competent authority. However, Article 3 of the Directive states:

'The provisions of this Directive shall not affect the powers of the Member States' authorities either as regards the setting of prices for medicinal products or their inclusion in the scope of national health insurance schemes on the basis of health, economic and social conditions'.

The 'limited list'

In the UK the first real intervention in the exercise of clinical judgement by doctors arose in 1985 with the introduction of the 'limited list', subsequently given the politically more neutral name 'selected list'. The then Conservative Government isolated seven therapeutic categories, principally concerned with what were viewed as more 'trivial' conditions, and put out for consultation a 'white list' of what it was proposed should continue to be prescribable; the balance of the products in those categories were to be 'black-listed'. Until this time, any product that was authorised for marketing would automatically be reimbursable if prescribed. Under paragraph 43 of their terms of service (Schedule 2 of the NHS (General Medical Services) Regulations 1992), doctors could 'order any drugs or appliances which are needed for the treatment of any patient ... by issuing a prescription' in the prescribed form. However, legislation in 1985 amended the contract with general practitioners so that this obligation was subject to paragraph 44, which reads as follows:

> 'A doctor shall not order ... a drug specified in Schedule 10 or Schedule 11 ... but may otherwise prescribe such a drug or other substance for that patient in the course of that treatment'.

A parallel change was made to the terms of service governing pharmacists (Schedule 2 of the NHS (Pharmaceutical Services) Regulations 1992), who were henceforth forbidden from dispensing on the NHS a product that had been black-listed. Schedule 10 was created to contain the names of products that could not be prescribed at all – most were branded products where a generic equivalent existed and was available at lower cost. Products were added to Schedule 11 where they were viewed as cost-effective for certain of their indications but not for others. A prescription for such a product had to be endorsed by the doctor as falling within the exception allowing prescription in Schedule 11. At the same time, the Government took the opportunity to give statutory force to the advice of the ACBS by including 'borderline products' in the black list or (as appropriate) in Schedule 11 (sometimes called the 'grey list').

It was argued (with considerable justification) that the creation of the black list did not inhibit doctors from meeting all real clinical needs with products still prescribable on the NHS. If, despite the NHS being capable of meeting that need more cheaply, a patient insisted upon having a product that was black-listed, the final words of paragraph 44 allowed the doctor to prescribe that product privately. Although the change in the text did not change the law that no charge could be made for the private prescription, the patient would pay the pharmacist for the dispensing of the product privately. It will be seen in the context of how doctors will be affected by the recommendations of NICE that, unless a product is black-listed, it is outside a doctor's powers to prescribe privately to a patient on his NHS list.

When the amendment was made to paragraph 44, it was implicitly on the basis that there would never be a situation where the NHS was unable to provide a product that would meet the patient's clinical need just as well as others that might be more expensive (but not more effective). This was reflected in the terms of reference of the Advisory Committee on NHS Drugs (ACD), which was established to advise the Secretary of State on which drugs within the seven therapeutic categories should be added to Schedule 10 or Schedule 11. The ACD was a non-statutory body but had appointed to it scientists and doctors with the necessary qualifications to assess what products were needed to meet all real clinical needs but at the lowest price. It was said by the then Minister of Health that it approached its task on the following basis:

> '... was the product required to satisfy a real clinical or therapeutic need not met as effectively by any other product available? If so, it was put on the list regardless of cost. Secondly, did it meet a real clinical need at least as effectively and at the same price as or more cheaply than any other available product? If so, it too was put on the list. Any products that were more expensive but not more effective were excluded'.[3]

The same statement noted that the ACD took a wide view of the components of clinical need. The assessment criteria were said to require consideration:

> '... not only of the specific therapeutic action of the products but also such problems as the acceptability and palatability of the products – especially for children, old people and the dying – and the need to have a choice of effective remedies wherever practicable'.

The administrative machinery for reaching decisions was contentious at first but by 1993 was relatively precise (ACD 1993) and generally acceptable to industry. As part of the machinery for making assessments, manufacturers were invited to make representations to the ACD which would then develop a provisional decision and notify this to the manufacturer in question. The manufacturer would then have the opportunity to make further representations and, in appropriate cases, would have an oral hearing before the Committee, before a final recommendation was made to the Secretary of State. It was only from 1993 that the right of other persons affected by the decision (e.g. professional groups and patients) to make representations was fully recognised. Ministers announced that they would make known the changes proposed to the black list about one month before the relevant statutory instrument was laid. This period of advance notification was also said to take account of the fact that any order is laid before Parliament for 21 days before it comes into force but in practice, of course, by this stage a complainant's ability to persuade ministers to make amendments has to be viewed as much reduced (DoH 1993a).

---

3.   The Rt. Hon. Kenneth Clarke, MP, *Hansard* 5 March 1985.

In 1992, the 'limited list' was extended to a further ten therapeutic categories that now went well beyond what could be categorised as trivial conditions. In the face of concerns expressed both by the medical profession and by the pharmaceutical industry, the Secretary of State continued to emphasise that 'a full range of other products remains available on the NHS so that patients will continue to receive all the medicines they need' (ibid.).

The operation of the concept of the 'limited list' in these new therapeutic areas was not without its difficulties. The conditions and the treatment options were much more complicated and, despite its terms of references which appeared to postulate no intervention in pricing and reimbursement where a product was found to offer therapeutic advantages over another, the ACD did seek to establish a form of reference pricing within some categories. A basic price was suggested and improvements in efficacy and safety over the benchmark product were subjectively valued, with the Committee proposing a price premium above the benchmark product price that was often less than the manufacturer's existing price. In the light of the ACD's terms of reference, many companies resisted such price fixing. It will be interesting to see how, with its wider terms of reference, NICE will deal with cost differentials within a therapeutic class.

The Secretary of State also faced difficulties in 1993 when products for nicotine replacement therapy were first authorised under the Medicines Act. This therapeutic field was not within the 17 categories over which the ACD had jurisdiction and, as it was classed and assessed as a medicine, it was surprising when the ACBS proposed its black-listing. That step was subsequently accepted by the Department of Health to be outside the jurisdiction of the ACBS but at the time the controversy was resolved when the products, which had initially been classed as prescription-only, were reclassified as 'pharmacy-only'. The availability of a product over the counter has been declared by the European Court to be a proper basis for the health schemes of Member States refusing to reimburse, although Dr Brian Mawhinney, Minister for Health, justified the exclusion on a more populist basis saying: 'People who can afford to smoke can also afford to buy products which may help them to stop smoking' (DoH 1993b).

Transparency of decision-making

In this context it should be noted that European law has intervened only to the extent of requiring Member States to adopt a transparent decision-making process. Partly as a result of the UK Government's initiative in introducing the 'limited list' in 1985, the European Commission issued a Communication (86/C310/08) in 1986 which set out some ground rules relating to the provision of reasons and proper appeal rights. In 1989, with increasing concern about the approach of several Member States to these sensitive issues, the Commission proposed a Directive which was adopted in the same year as the Transparency Directive (89/105/EEC). This provided that any decision to exclude a product from coverage under a national health scheme must be based on a statement of reasons, using objective and verifiable criteria that had been published nationally and notified to the European Commission. The decisions and reasoning, including expert opinions upon which they were based, were to be made available and affected manufacturers were to be informed of the remedies available to them in law and the time allowed for pursuing those remedies. The Directive relates to medicines but its principles are generally applicable to other interventions, such as medical devices, as the aim is to ensure fair treatment of persons affected and to avoid unjustifiable hindrances to the free movement of goods. European law does not, however, currently provide substantive assistance to patients demanding treatment under the NHS.

Further challenges by patients and manufacturers

The 1990s saw an increase in the willingness of patients to challenge the refusal of health authorities (themselves under increasing financial pressures) to provide access to many of the newer and more expensive treatments. Once more, however, the courts showed themselves reluctant to intervene, except in the most exceptional cases. Accordingly, when Cambridge Health Authority refused to underwrite expensive experimental treatment for a child with leukaemia, when those treating the child thought the intervention had a limited chance of success and could not properly be justified, the court indicated that it would not substitute its judgement for that of the clinicians in charge of the patient:

'I have no doubt that in a perfect world any treatment which a patient, or a patient's family, sought would be provided if doctors were willing to give it, no matter how much it cost, particularly when a life was potentially at stake. It would however, in my view, be shutting one's eyes to the real world if the court were to proceed on the basis that we do live in such a world. It is common knowledge that health authorities of all kinds are constantly pressed to make ends meet. They cannot pay their nurses as much as they would like; they cannot provide all the treatments they would like; they cannot purchase all the extremely expensive medical equipment they would like; they cannot carry out all the research they would like; they cannot build all the hospitals and specialist units they would like. Difficult and agonising judgements have to be made as to how a limited budget is best allocated to the maximum advantage to the maximum number of patients. That is not a judgement which the court can make'.[4]

More recently still, the Court of Appeal has again emphasised that the obligation of the Secretary of State under Section 1 of the NHS Act to provide a 'comprehensive' health service and to secure the effective provision of services in the prevention, diagnosis and treatment of illness, is qualified. The judgment of the court in *R v North and East Devon Health Authority,* ex parte *Coughlan* (1999) makes it clear that not all services

---

4.   Sir Thomas Bingham in *R* v *Cambridge Health Authority*, ex parte *B* (1995) 1 WLR 898.

have to be provided if the Secretary of State considers that they are not reasonably required or are not a necessary adjunct to a requirement itself judged reasonable.

Where the families of haemophiliacs challenged the refusal of the relevant health authorities to fund treatment with the recombinant product – preferred by their doctors for its viral safety – on the grounds that effective but cheaper products existed, the court refused permission even to bring the case (while not excluding the possibility that certain exceptional cases might justify use of the more expensive product) (*R* v *East Lancashire Health Authority,* ex parte *B and others* 1997).

Manufacturers who sought to challenge the Secretary of State in respect of the exclusion of particular products from reimbursement fared no better. In 1996 the company Scherer challenged the decision of the Secretary of State to exclude from NHS prescription capsules of temazepam. The capsules had been associated with misuse by addicts and alternatives (of tablets) for legitimate medical purposes remained prescribable. The Secretary of State acted upon the recommendation of the Advisory Council on the Misuse of Drugs by black-listing the capsules (DoH 1995b), and the court refused to accept that the decision was outside his powers. It stated that cost having regard to the availability of equally effective alternatives was not the only basis for exclusion, although it was accepted that hitherto that had been the basic approach adopted by successive governments. It emphasised once again the broad discretion that the Secretary of State possessed, subject only to him not being entitled to exercise his powers in a way that denied patients 'adequate care and attendance' (*R* v *Secretary of State for Health,* ex parte *R P Scherer Ltd* 1996).

The courts have made it clear, however, that they will intervene where policy guidelines are issued by the Secretary of State and these are ignored completely on cost grounds. The introduction of new classes of drugs to treat serious illnesses has increasingly been accompanied by the provision of advice from SMAC and/or the NHS Executive endorsed by the Secretary of State.

The Department of Health took this approach when providing advice on the use of beta-interferons in the treatment of multiple sclerosis. General advice was given, although not in a way that compromised clinical freedom:

> *'If authorisation is granted, the drug will – in line with the commitment of Ministers that patients should receive the treatments which they clinically need – become available for NHS prescription, subject to any conditions which may be attached to the marketing authorisations and to clinical decisions about the appropriateness of treatment in individual cases'* (NHS Executive 1995).

Where, despite the promulgation of this guidance, North Derbyshire Health Authority developed its own guidelines that effectively excluded treatment on cost grounds, the court ruled the Authority's approach illegal: 'A blanket ban was the very antithesis of national policy, whose aim was to target the drug appropriately at patients who were most likely to benefit from treatment' (*R* v *North Derbyshire Health Authority,* ex parte *Fisher* 1997).

In so doing the court had regard to the sentiments expressed in January 1996 by the then Secretary of State, Stephen Dorrell:

> *'There should be no clinically effective treatment which a health authority decides as a matter of principle should not be provided: there will always be the exceptional case where treatment is clinically justified. To ban treatment in such circumstances would be inconsistent with the principles upon which the NHS is established and I do not believe that they represent acceptable practice'.*[5]

With the change in Government in 1997 few anticipated that the new Secretary of State would himself ban an innovative new product from prescription in the way that occurred on the introduction of Viagra (sildenafil). Inevitably, the case ended up in the courts.

The Viagra litigation

Viagra represented the first licensed oral treatment for erectile dysfunction. It was an innovative and highly effective product authorised by the European authorities following a centralised application (allowing, if granted, marketing in all Member States) and it was judged by the Committee for Proprietary Medicinal Products within the European Medicines Evaluation Agency (EMEA) as suitable for prescription by general practitioners and not just by consultants. When it reached the market, it was cheaper than the pre-existing medicinal and non-medicinal interventions. It was outside the existing jurisdiction of the ACD and ACBS but health authorities were expressing concerns about the potential effect on their budgets if no restriction upon reimbursement was imposed. Mr Frank Dobson, the Secretary of State at the time, authorised the issue of a Circular advising doctors that they should not prescribe Viagra until further notice and that health authorities should not support provision 'other than in exceptional circumstances which they should require be cleared in advance with them' (DoH 1998).

General practitioners were placed in a very difficult position. Most rightly assumed that they had an obligation to treat patients according to their clinical judgement as to each patient's needs but on the other hand they were put under very great pressure by their health authorities to abide by the contents of the Circular. Some health authorities expressly stated that they could not foresee any 'exceptional circumstances' (see notice from South and West Devon Health Authority of 15 September 1998). Some health authorities went so far as to say that they would 'take measures to recover all costs from the prescriber' if the advice was contravened (see Isle of Wight Health Authority notice to general practitioners of 9 October 1998). There was, in fact, no statutory basis for such recovery under the NHS legislation.

The dilemma for doctors was increased by the fact that the statutory machinery for legitimate black-listing of a product had not been operated and, therefore, strictly

---

5. The Rt. Hon. Stephen Dorrell MP, The Millennium Lecture, 8 January 1996.

speaking, there was no basis within the law for prescribing privately to a patient on the doctor's NHS list. This would only be legitimate if the product was black-listed, whereupon the words of paragraph 44 of the terms of service would be triggered ('but may otherwise prescribe such a drug ... for that patient'). Some doctors ignored this impediment and prescribed privately; others referred patients to a different practice for private prescription. Although the initial Health Circular had anticipated the ban being overtaken within a few weeks by definitive advice from SMAC on the place of Viagra in the treatment of erectile dysfunction, SMAC's deliberations took longer than the Secretary of State expected. Even when they became available in November 1998, they did not provide a justification for black-listing. On the contrary, they were generally supportive of the ability of general practitioners to diagnose erectile dysfunction and prescribe the product in appropriate cases. While stating that Government would have to make the decision on whether the resource implications were consistent with priorities within the NHS, SMAC emphasised the need for equality of access for all patients with the condition, whatever its cause.

It was not until 21 January 1999 that the Secretary of State announced a public consultation exercise on proposals that would restrict prescription of Viagra (and now all other licensed treatments) to limited classes of patients whose erectile dysfunction was due to specified underlying circumstances. For the first time, it was proposed that prescription should not be on the basis of real clinical need but rather by reference to whether the cause of that need fell within one of a limited number of underlying conditions or causes. For other men suffering from erectile dysfunction, it was proposed that treatment should be available only in 'exceptional circumstances' after specialist assessment in a hospital.The Secretary of State made it clear that his decision to discriminate between the causes of erectile dysfunction was cost-related:

'Now that the treatment is available in tablet form, the cost of treating impotence could escalate. The cost could increase ten-fold or even more. To limit this impact, we propose controls which reflect the priority given to treatment for impotence, and reflect its current level of expenditure' (DoH 1999a).

Consistent with this, the Government took steps to change the main criterion which hitherto had determined exclusion from prescription, namely the cost of a product, having regard to the alternative products available that met the same clinical need as effectively. On 16 February 1999 the European Commission was notified by the UK Government of new terms of reference for reimbursement decisions under the NHS. Although the catalyst for this change was the Viagra controversy, the new terms of reference have general application and give the Secretary of State a much wider basis upon which to black-list products consequent upon the advice of NICE. The principal provisions read as follows:

'A medicinal product or a category of medicinal products may be excluded entirely from supply on NHS prescription. It may alternatively be excluded except in specified circumstances, or except in relation to specified conditions or categories of condition, or specified categories of patient. The medicinal product or a category of them may be so excluded where the forecast aggregate cost to the NHS of allowing the product (or category of products) to be supplied on NHS prescription, or to be supplied more widely than the permitted exceptions, could not be justified having regard to all the relevant circumstances including in particular the Secretary of State's duties pursuant to the NHS Act 1977 and the priorities for expenditure of NHS resources'. [6]

The terms of reference, therefore, expressly sanction the restriction of prescription to particular categories of patients where those categories are designed to ensure that costs to the NHS do not exceed a particular pre-existing level or level judged acceptable, even if higher. As such, this allowed the Secretary of State so to construct the categories of patients for whom erectile dysfunction treatments could be prescribed that the overall level of expenditure on erectile dysfunction would not exceed materially the amount spent before Viagra was authorised. The fact that some of the commonest causes of erectile dysfunction were excluded meant for the first time that there would be discrimination between patients upon factors other than clinical need. Unsurprisingly, the British Medical Association (BMA) expressed strong criticism of the Secretary of State's proposed decision. Although the Secretary of State had said that until the consultation was complete and a final decision made, doctors should not prescribe Viagra on the NHS, the General Practitioners Committee (GPC) of the BMA issued a policy statement that general practitioners should, where clinically appropriate, continue to prescribe Viagra, unless and until the law was changed.

In the meantime, however, Pfizer Limited, the market authorisation holder for Viagra, had taken their own action to test the legality of the ban instituted by the Secretary of State. Judicial review proceedings were commenced in December 1998 and on 26 May 1999 Mr Justice Collins ruled that the ban implicit in the original Health Circular was illegal. In so doing, he clarified the obligations of general practitioners under their terms of service. The Health Circular was found to be illegal both under domestic law and under European law. As to domestic law, the court found that the GP's obligation in treating patients under the NHS was to render all necessary and appropriate services according to clinical judgement, subject only to the statutory obligation not to prescribe a product that had been black-listed in accordance with the existing legislation. In this case the court noted that Viagra had not been black-listed but the 'guidance' was couched as a ban and had clearly been intended to act as a ban:

'To state in bald terms that Viagra should not be prescribed save in (undefined) exceptional circumstances is tantamount to telling the recipients

6. Written Answers: *Hansard* 28 June 1999 Medicines Selected List Scheme: Exclusions at WA9.

of the advice to follow it. They cannot know how their professional judgement should be influenced by the advice. In my judgement, the evidence confirms that this was and was intended to be acted upon by GPs independently of whether in their professional judgement a patient needed treatment for ED and so should have the better treatment available, namely Viagra. Thus I am satisfied that the Circular was and is unlawful in terms of domestic law' (*R* v *Secretary of State for Health,* ex parte *Pfizer Ltd* 1999).

The Secretary of State had argued that the initiative did not involve a ban and, being guidance only, did not require compliance with the Transparency Directive. The court disagreed and dealt with the matter relatively shortly:

'The Directive sets out requirements (and domestic law to the same effect) which are to be complied with before the black-listing of a product can take place. It cannot be correct to bypass those requirements, which are there to safeguard the applicant's rights, and to restrict the product's marketing without complying with them'.

On this basis, a breach of Community law was found as well.

The decision, while important both in relation to the obligations of doctors and in relation to the Secretary of State's powers when faced with similar issues, did not preclude the Secretary of State restricting the availability of Viagra through the operation of the proper machinery. On 7 May 1999, the Friday before the Monday on which the application came before the court, the Secretary of State announced[7] that he proposed to make regulations on 1 July 1999 to limit the prescription of all treatments for erectile dysfunction on the NHS to men who suffered it as a result of various specified causes (a slightly expanded list to that proposed with the original consultation paper) or who were receiving treatment (which, of course, would have been other than with Viagra) before Viagra was authorised on 14 September 1998. This was achieved by adding the product to Schedule 11 and the black-listing also legitimised private prescriptions by NHS doctors (provided no change was made).

The decision has considerable implications for the manner in which the Secretary of State reacts to the judgements of NICE. Based on the advice of NICE, he may issue (or encourage NICE to issue) advice to doctors indicating in strong terms that he considers it undesirable that they prescribe a particular product or prescribe it for a particular type of patient, but the final decision whether to prescribe a product that has not been black-listed lies with the doctor concerned. Alternatively, the Secretary of State must translate the advice of NICE into a formal proposal to black-list.

---

7. DoH Statement of 7 May (1999/0274) and NHS (General Medical Services) Amendment No 2 Regulations SI 1999 No 1627.

The National Institute for Clinical Excellence

NICE was created as a Special Health Authority as of 26 February 1999 with such functions in connection with the promotion of clinical excellence as the Secretary of State may direct.[8] The functions are described as 'to appraise the clinical benefits and the costs of those interventions notified by the Secretary of State and to make recommendations'. The recommendations are to focus upon whether the intervention in question can be recommended as a cost-effective use of NHS resources either generally or for specific indications and whether for all patients or defined sub-groups, and whether as first-line or second-line treatment. The recommendations may describe the further research needed before relevant questions can be answered adequately. The Institute is expected to take steps to ensure that the final guidance is reflected in clinical guidelines on the subject, in PRODIGY guidelines, and in other protocols and material prepared by the NHS for use by its relevant bodies and services.

At the same time regulations came into force[9] concerning its constitution. NICE consists of a chairman (currently, Professor Sir Michael Rawlins), seven members who are not office holders (all appointed by the Secretary of State) and four other office holders, who must include a Chief Officer, Chief Finance Officer and Clinical Director, all appointed by the Institute itself (subject in the case of the Chief Officer (Chief Executive) to the approval of the Secretary of State).

Under Regulation 9, in accordance with Directions given by the Secretary of State, the all-important Appraisal Committee is appointed by the Institute. The standing members were announced in September 1999 (NICE 1999b) with Professor David Barnett as chairman of the Committee with the remit to advise the Board of the Institute on such matters about which the Board seeks guidance and in particular:

'... the use, within the NHS, of any new or established health technology in relation to its clinical and cost-effectiveness taking into account the interests of the service as a whole'.

Members are appointed for three years and up to five specific experts may be co-opted for particular reviews. The membership is diverse and includes 21 persons (including the Chairman) with a wide range of expertise from general medicine to pathology, biostatistics and surgery. There are places for, among others, general practitioners, health economists, nurses, pharmacists, patient advocates and health managers. Where data relating to new and advanced technologies are under review, it seems likely that the Committee will rely for significant aspects of the appraisal on co-opted specialists.

In August 1999, NICE issued interim guidance (NICE 1999a) for manufacturers on how assessments would take place. The Guidance states that all the clinical benefits of an intervention will be assessed, including effects on quality of life as well as effects on mortality and these will be set against estimates of the associated costs. In reaching its judgement NICE is asked to have regard to certain factors listed in the

8. The National Institute for Clinical Excellence (Establishment and Constitution) Order SI 1999 No 220.
9. The National Institute for Clinical Excellence Regulations SI 1999 No 260.

Secretary of State's Directions, which are said to include the Secretary of State's clinical priorities; the degree of clinical need of patients with a particular condition (the draft July Guidance referred to 'the expectation of the quality and length of life of patients in the absence of the intervention under consideration); the broad balance of benefits and costs; the effective use of available resources and any guidance from the Secretary of State on the resources likely to be available. The Guidance also states that NICE will be 'sympathetic' to the longer-term interest of the NHS in encouraging innovations provided they are 'of good value to patients' – this last phrase was added after consultation on the draft of July 1999 which was published.

The Department of Health determines which interventions are referred to NICE following consultation with interested parties and the Institute itself. The aim is that referral will take place at least nine months (amended from 12 months in the July draft) before the date by which it is intended that the Guidance be disseminated. For pharmaceuticals it is said that notification should coincide with the submission for marketing authorisation. The intention is said to be that guidance should be available to the NHS as soon as possible after launch or general dissemination of the technology. This is important because, as the NHS legislation is currently drafted, products are reimbursable automatically upon a marketing authorisation being granted, unless and until any 'black-listing' becomes effective. Black-listing takes time because it involves amendment to Schedules to the relevant NHS Regulations, through the laying of the appropriate Statutory Instrument. For established technologies, submissions are expected within three months of notification of review.

The timetable for assessment of particular interventions has clearly been developed to ensure an adequate timetable for representations from manufacturers be considered and to ensure that other interested parties (essentially patient and professional groups) have the opportunity to make representations. The timetable from submission of evidence to guidance from NICE is expected to be six months but it is not entirely clear how this timetable can be met where the approved indications are contentious and the details are not known until shortly before an authorisation is granted.

The Chief Executive noted in July 1999 that members may ask NICE to undertake a rapid assessment. Although this is said not to be a substitute for the formal appraisal process, the effect of the recommendations of NICE (even if only on an interim basis) will be just as significant and there must be potential for concertinered time-lines resulting in an assessment that falls short of the declared aim of achieving 'a transparent and well-structured process' that ensures adequate time to make submissions and a fair opportunity to comment upon draft conclusions.

Appraisal criteria

The appraisal criteria against which data are to be submitted are said by the August Guidance to be: clinical effectiveness; cost-effectiveness; and the wider NHS implications.

In relation to clinical effectiveness this is said to encompass 'actual or projected benefits' which may include 'reductions in morbidity or mortality, improved quality of life, or other measures of positive outcome'. Both qualitative and quantitative aspects will be considered for all patients and for sub-groups, with particular attention being given to the times at which clinical outcomes were assessed. Quantitative comparisons with other forms of treatment are to be provided. As the regulatory process has hitherto focused upon proof of efficacy invariably using placebo-controlled clinical trials, the lack of 'head-to-head' data, where the comparator is the current standard therapy, may prove unhelpful to manufacturers, although model comparisons based upon published literature are suggested as an alternative. In relation to endpoints used in trials and, in particular, quality of life, the Guidance notes the need to model the data so as to relate the conclusions to UK conditions. Longer term, there surely will be a cost implication in the development of increasingly sophisticated data from studies with sufficient power to identify differences either generally or in sub-groups. The cost will be passed on in the price of medicines.

In relation to cost-effectiveness the Guidance endorses the standard approaches of cost minimisation, cost utility, cost benefit and cost-effectiveness. In the consideration of costs, both direct and indirect costs (including costs to both the primary and secondary care sectors and to the Personal Social Services) are said to be relevant. The wider costs and benefits (including allowing patients to return to gainful employment) may be addressed but the discrete costs to the NHS must always be transparent. For these purposes as part of the conclusion on the wider NHS implications, data on the likely number of eligible patients for the intervention are to be presented. It is said that NICE accepts that at this stage manufacturers may not be able to provide full information of the type required to make an optimal evaluation.

The original discussion paper relating to NICE (NHS Executive 1999a) noted the need to avoid 'placing disproportionate burdens on those who are developing clinical innovations for use in the NHS or risking delay in the effective introduction of those innovations offering worldwide benefits to patients'. Industry was reassured that Government said that NICE would not hold companies to the impossible task of satisfying criteria where the relevant data could not reasonably have been produced:

'Transitional arrangements will be needed over the next few years, in particular for medicines, since any clinical research needed to satisfy the licensing requirements will already be underway. Under these circumstances it would be unreasonable to require information which was not obtainable from the research already underway, since that would imply new research and might delay, perhaps by several years, the launch of the product. We believe that this would be unrealistic for many companies, especially those with international markets'.

Longer term, the development of detailed data of the type being sought by NICE not only carries a cost implication but also seems to presuppose that the product has already been the subject of extensive post-research use. Indeed, there are many examples of products whose most significant benefits only became apparent in the years after first marketing (the ACE inhibitors and the taxanes are but two examples). The Association of the British Pharmaceutical Industry (ABPI) has expressed grave reservations about the potential impact upon innovation and the attractions of the UK market as a place to research and to plan to launch innovative new products:

> 'Realistic health economic evaluation cannot be made until the product has been in widespread use for a number of years, and further delaying entry into the NHS would have a negative impact on health care services and be a disservice to patients' (ABPI 1999).

The ABPI suggested that initially there be no recommendation against use (although guidance could indicate the areas where further research was needed for a full appraisal) until after a full appraisal had taken place, which would be after an agreed period of time from launch (depending upon the nature and size of the patient population in issue). This is not the way in which NICE is to operate but it will not be possible to judge whether ABPI's concerns are well-founded until the experience of NICE assessments is greater. Clearly, industry did not feel reassured by the fast-track appraisal of Glaxo Wellcome's new influenza product, Relenza (zanamivir), which received a negative assessment in October 1999 (NICE 1999c). This was only a preliminary assessment with a full assessment due in 2000.

Evaluation

Submissions made by manufacturers and others are evaluated by the Secretariat of NICE or designated outside groups, which may seek additional information from manufacturers. The Secretariat prepares an evaluation report and a draft provisional determination for consideration by the Appraisal Committee. It would seem, therefore, that the evaluation reports are likely to be very influential. The expertise of the outside groups which NICE is likely to rely upon will be critical particularly in the early stages of the work of NICE when the Appraisal Committee will be under pressure to review many interventions over a relatively short time period.

The timetable envisages the Appraisal Committee having the report about four weeks prior to its appraisal meeting. The process of assessment follows a similar course to that adopted by the ACD under the 'selected list' initiative. The Committee may invite oral representations from manufacturers as part of its consideration of the submissions made and the report and draft provisional determination. The Head of Appraisals is responsible for ensuring that the report is assembled properly and the provisional determination is prepared. He receives the submission and must ensure that the report and draft determination are available not more than 12 weeks thereafter.

The provisional determination is released to manufacturers and other interested parties with the report (redacted as to commercially confidential information when sent to third parties). It will contain the provisional conclusions and proposed guidance to the NHS together with information on the clinical audit method appropriate for monitoring adherence to the guidance. The manufacturer is then allowed a period of about four weeks within which to consider the draft proposals before the Committee reconsiders its provisional determination and submits a final opinion to the Board of NICE. The Board then forwards it in confidence to the manufacturer, who has ten days to decide whether to appeal to the Board against the conclusions of the Committee. Appeals are to be heard within 28 days by three non-executive Board members and two independent members. However, the Guidance does not appear to contemplate a meaningful appeal on the merits but rather only submissions as to procedural fairness (unless the appeal is based on the contention that the decision is perverse on its face). Consistent with this any new data submitted will normally be referred back to the Committee and the hearing adjourned pending its assessment.

In December 1999 the Government announced that the regulations governing NICE would be amended to require it, when carrying out its functions, to take account of 'the effective use of available resources'. This change is viewed by many as encouraging NICE to make recommendations not on the basis of a scientific assessment of 'cost-effectiveness' relative to other products available for the same condition but on the wholly subjective issue of 'affordability', which has a political dimension. The change is entirely consistent with the change in the terms of reference for reimbursement in the UK notified by the Secretary of State to the European Commission in February 1999 and some would argue that medical advisers should not be insulated from the need to provide advice that has proper regard to resource issues. However, SMAC's advice of 9 November 1998 on Viagra seems to indicate the understandable reluctance of the profession to mix medical questions with political ones, at least where no proper financial framework has been set by Government:

'(i) SMAC recognises that the aim of prescribing sildenafil is to correct the distressing condition of erectile dysfunction so that sexual function returns towards normal. In common with many treatments available under the NHS this improves quality of life, but does not save or prolong it.

*(ii) Provided that sildenafil is prescribed only to patients who have the medical condition of erectile dysfunction, SMAC sees no **medical** reason why it should not be available on the NHS in accordance with the terms of the summary of product characteristics in the marketing authorisation; nor why it should not be prescribed by GPs with referral to hospital specialists where appropriate.*

(iii) SMAC suggests that Ministers should consider the priority to be given to all methods of managing erectile dysfunction within the NHS relative to treatments for other conditions, but that any decision takes into account equity of access as well as availability of resources. Doctors will need clear Government support and national guidance.

(iv) Once Ministers have decided in principle on the prescribing of sildenafil, SMAC would be happy if so requested to prepare appropriate clinical guidance for doctors'.

In Parliament, ministers have said that the change in the declared function of NICE by the Department's lawyers was recommended in the light of the Viagra experience. The remit of the Appraisal Committee of NICE will clearly, therefore, be much wider than that of SMAC or the ACD.

Enforcement

The functions of NICE are likely to be closely interlinked with those of the Commission for Health Improvement (CHI), created by Section 17 of the Health Act 1999, which is to provide advice and to audit the quality of health care provided through health authorities. The extent to which 'clinical governance' (see Miles *et al.* 2000) will become a byword for taking steps to challenge any deviation from the advice of NICE remains to be seen but, in determining the significance of a change of policy, the level of enforcement of that policy is often more important in practice than the policy itself (see Chapter 9 of this volume). The Chairman of NICE has indicated that he expects doctors to follow NICE's recommendations closely (Anon 1999a). It would seem that deviation from the NICE view will have to be justified. However, the fact that NICE is in principle advisory only is very clear. This has been emphasised by ministers in Parliament: [10]

'The intention is that the National Institute will issue authoritative guidance to health professionals ...'

'NICE will provide that information, but NICE has no power to determine what decision is taken in each individual case. If a drug or treatment were ruled out on the NHS, that could only be by the Government, and therefore by Ministers, as is the case at present'.

The option of translating the judgements of NICE into black-listing of products clearly remains:

'If, having read NICE guidance, Ministers concluded that it should be enforced by regulation, it must remain the responsibility of Ministers to take such a decision ...'.

10. Mr Alan Milburn, Minister of Health, *Hansard* 15 June 1999

Private health care alternatives

One difficulty is that if the Secretary of State seeks to rely upon the general authority of NICE and its ability to define 'quality' in relation to prescribing decisions without the need for black-listing, manufacturers could face a situation where the development of a private market is effectively excluded because, as has been seen, in the absence of black-listing, it will not be legal for a doctor to prescribe privately to a patient on that doctor's NHS list. The restrictions banning private prescription are understandable when all clinical needs can be met by products available on the NHS, but when they are not (as is transparently the case in relation to treatments for erectile dysfunction, multiple sclerosis and – some would say – schizophrenia and cancer) patients' freedom of choice and convenience are severely infringed, if they cannot opt to pay their doctor for private treatment. Even with black-listing, patients cannot be charged for the service of giving a prescription privately or for supplying the medicine itself.[11]

Moreover, if partial black-listing takes place pursuant to Schedule 11 in a way that arbitrarily excludes certain patients from treatment under the NHS because of the cost implications of allowing all patients with the same clinical need to be treated, questions must surely be raised as to whether this is the fairest method of allocating limited financial resources. It would perhaps be fairer to institute a system of co-payment of the type common within the European Community under which, in appropriate cases, all patients with the same clinical need will receive some support rather than some receiving completely free treatment and others receiving no treatment at all (unless they can pay for private treatment). A co-payment system would perhaps also involve less disruption of the marketplace. In the UK, where over 90 per cent of prescriptions are on the NHS, the black-listing of a product reduces enormously the market for that product there, which may have a major effect on trade between Member States. The possibility of the NHS Executive giving strong advice against NHS prescription but without black-listing a product may be worse; the pharmaceutical company could find its NHS market removed and its ability to create a private market even more severely circumscribed. Recently, Merck Sharpe & Dohme invited the Department to black-list its new medicinal product for baldness (Anon 1999b). At the same time, the BMA noted the increasing concern of GPs about their inability to charge for the consulting time involved in providing private prescriptions.

Conclusion

It seems likely that the creation of NICE represents merely one step in the process whereby the Government will seek to ensure more consistency in the use of resources within different parts of the NHS. Certainly that aim is to be applauded. The level of postcode prescribing of medicines such as beta-interferons and the obfuscation of health authorities in relation to funding issues has become a national disgrace. Admittedly, authorities have often been put in impossible positions because of the mismatch between their allocated funding and the demands on them. The declared

---

11. See NHS Executive Circular HSC 1999/148 of 30 June 1999 for a discussion of what can and cannot be done privately under the legislation once a product has been black-listed.

aims of NICE in relation to equity of access deserve support, although some fear that NICE will in practice merely regularise reduced access to the more expensive and innovative medicines (see, for instance, Ellis 1998).

On any view NICE has an unenviable task. The difficulties it will face in applying objectively rather nebulous criteria to produce judgements that are essentially subjective are probably insurmountable, unless the process is part of a wider public debate upon treatment priorities. This must entail a review of support across all therapeutic areas and not just the new technologies. The process at present potentially discriminates against innovation by allowing insufficient time to make a proper assessment of the risks and benefits of that innovation.

Most importantly, there is need for a much more sophisticated and open political debate about the available resources against which these different decisions are to be made. Editorial comment in the national press is increasingly pressing for that debate in ever more emotive language – one national paper has spoken of the NHS 'rotting before our eyes, with a lack of political will to make the tough choices for a first class service for an ever more demanding population'(Anon 2000). It is certainly ironic that in the same month as NICE was created and one month before the announcement of the cost-driven decision on restriction of prescription of Viagra, the Secretary of State, Frank Dobson, reiterated the continued adherence to the 1948 principles and the supremacy of the doctor as ultimate decision-maker:

> *'The Government is absolutely committed to the fundamental rule that the NHS is there to provide services for everybody on the basis of clinical need ... The responsibility for deciding what treatment is best for the patient rests with the doctors concerned, in consultation with the patient, informed by the patient's clinical history. These decisions are frequently complex and may need to take account of a range of factors; chief among these must be the ability of any patient to benefit from any proposed treatment'* (DoH 1999b).

While the political rhetoric continues in this vein, NICE will have an uphill battle in getting acceptance of its efforts to provide an answer to the basic problems posed by a scheme that continues to aim for 'clinical excellence', while refusing to confront the cost of achieving it in today's environment. Nevertheless, it deserves wholehearted support in trying to make progress in a field critical to a variety of interests but, most importantly, the legitimate expectation of the population at large that it should benefit from the great improvements in public health that science is making possible.

References

[ABPI] The Association of the British Pharmaceutical Industry (1999). *NICE and medicines.* ABPI. BSC/6/99/4K.

[ACD] Advisory Committee on NHS Drugs (1993). *Notes on guidance to manufacturers.* ACD, Department of Health, London.

Anon (1965). *Report of the Standing Joint-Committee on Classification of Proprietary Preparations.* HMSO, London, para. 1.

Anon (1967). *Report on the definition of drugs (borderline substances).* Standing Joint-Committee on Classification of Proprietary Preparations. HMSO, London.

Anon (1997). *New Labour: because Britain deserves better.* The Labour Party M/029/97.

Anon (1999a). *Hospital Doctor* 19 August.

Anon (1999b). *Financial Times* 16 December.

Anon (2000). Brave new century [editorial]. *Sunday Times* 2 January.

DoH (1944). *A National Health Service* (Cmnd 6502). HMSO, London.

DoH (1993a). Press Release H93/895, 27 July.

DoH (1993b). Press Release H93/914, 12 August.

DoH (1995a). *The Patients' Charter and You.* Department of Health, London.

DoH (1995b). Press Release H95/382, 24 July.

DoH (1998). Health Service Circular 1998/158, 16 September.

DoH (1999a). Press Release 1999/0037, 21 January.

DoH (1999b). *NHS care for the elderly.* Press Release 1999/0241, 19 April 1999.

Ellis SJ (1998). Some unanswered questions about NICE. *J R Soc Med* **91**, 538–9.

Miles A, Hill A & Hurwitz B (2000). *Clinical governance: enabling excellence or imposing control?* Aesculapius Medical Press, London.

NHS Executive (1995). *New drugs for multiple sclerosis.* EL (95) 97. Leeds.

NHS Executive (1999a). *Faster access to modern treatment: how NICE appraisal will work.* Leeds, para. 7.

NHS Executive (1999b). Health Service Circular HSC 1999/148, 30 June.

NICE (1999a). *Appraisal of new and existing technologies: interim guidance for manufacturers and sponsors.* August 1999, 19A 050 899.

NICE (1999b). Press Release, 1999/006, 27 September.

NICE (1999c). *Rapid assessment – zanamivir (Relenza).* Press Release (1999/05), 1 October.

R v *Cambridge Health Authority,* ex parte *B* (1995). 1 WLR 898.

R v *East Lancashire Health Authority*, ex parte *B and others* (1997). QBD 27 February 1997 (unreported).

R v *North and East Devon Health Authority,* ex parte *Coughlan* (1999). *The Times Law Reports* 20 July 1999.

R v *North Derbyshire Health Authority,* ex parte *Fisher* (1997). 8 Med L R 327.

R v *Northwest Lancashire Health Authority*, ex parte *G and others* (1999). Court of Appeal 29 July 1999. *The Times Law Report* 24 August 1999.

R v *Secretary of State for Health,* ex parte *Pfizer Ltd* (1999). Lloyds Rep Med 289.

R v *Secretary of State for Health,* ex parte *R P Scherer Ltd* (1996). QBD 8 March 1996 (unreported).

R v *Secretary of State for Social Services and others,* ex parte *Hincks* (1980). BMLR 93.

Chapter 9

The evolution of the audit society, its politics of control and the advent of CHI

Michael Power

Introduction

In 1999 the UK Government created two new bodies to oversee the quality of health care provision: the National Institute for Clinical Excellence (NICE) and the Commission for Health Improvement (CHI). The two bodies will formally relate to each other as standard setter and enforcer respectively, a division of labour which is used in other regulatory systems. Nevertheless, beyond these formalities, there is little knowledge of how these new organisations will actually function. On the one hand, many health professionals remain nervous about an initiative which may erode their professional judgement and undermine their morale; they perceive NICE and CHI as products of a politics of control and discipline, rather than as institutions that can secure real quality for patients (Charlton 1999; Smith 1999). On the other hand, enthusiasts for these reforms take as given the need to eradicate variations in clinical judgement, and associated variations in cost, by developing clear clinical guidelines and by enforcing their implementation (Horton 1999).

This chapter provides an outsider's commentary on these developments and seeks to place them in the broader context of the 'audit society' (Power 1994, 1999). There is considerable suggestive evidence about the likely functioning of NICE and CHI, and it is reasonable to predict that CHI will become more significant than its formal relationship with NICE suggests. The next section provides a brief account of the 'audit society' thesis, noting some of the criticisms of its general applicability to the field of clinical governance and clinical audit. Following this, CHI is considered directly and it is predicted that standards-based clinical audit will generate pathologies at the micro-level of clinical practice. Finally, two possible paths of development for CHI are considered. One leads paradoxically to mediocrity and not excellence, whereby NICE and CHI can be viewed as 'fatal remedies' (Sieber 1981). The other requires CHI and similar organisations to become reflexive about their operations by processing their own side-effects. The prospect for such 'reflexive' monitoring raises a number of important issues for the audit society.

An 'audit' society? The age of inspection?

In the 1980s the UK experienced an explosion of monitoring, evaluating and assessing activity; not only did new careers open up in many sectors for auditors, inspectors and checkers, but organisational agents also found themselves subject to increasing scrutiny and accountability for performance. However, while we might agree on the phenomenon in general terms, it remains contentious to characterise it as an 'audit society', since many of the monitoring and assessment activities are not 'audits' according to the financial audit model. By the late 1990s the emphasis at policy levels had also shifted from audit to quality, performance, excellence and inspection (Bowerman *et al.* 2000). Nevertheless, the 'audit society' remains a useful label for a far-reaching set of changes in organisational life. A number of reasons or causes can be suggested for these changes.

First, a serious fiscal crisis and funding shortfalls led to a shift in public sector management philosophy towards the so-called 'new public management' (Hood 1991), an assembly of techniques and procedures in the service of efficiency and cost-effectiveness. Management techniques and related ideas about organisational design were borrowed from the private sector as blueprints for reform, even though it was always clear that private sector organisations never themselves functioned according to these blueprints. In this way the public sector was to become more like the private sector than the private sector itself. An important innovation was the programme to stimulate competition by creating provider and purchaser organisations, notably in the field of health care. This innovation drove new demands and requirements for monitoring, both in the traditional sense of financial propriety and also with an explicit focus on cost-effectiveness and efficiency.

Second, there were some closely related innovations in the area of quality assurance for goods and services based on general quality standards, such as ISO 9000 and its variants. Monitoring systems to ensure quality of goods and services emerged as an important advisory area across the public and private sectors. These developments also heralded a more explicit regulatory emphasis on the quality of management systems as the basis for high-quality performance. Despite widespread concern that quality assurance models were more about the quality of systems than substantive performance itself, a certain style of auditing and control grew rapidly and became a widely diffused template for thinking about organisational improvement.

A third important driver of the audit society has been an increasingly vociferous politics of transparency and accountability to stakeholders. At first, this took the form of 'value for money' for taxpayers, but the reference point changed over time to 'customers', the users of public services. Interestingly, *real* customers, such as patients, tend to have scant representation in the changes conducted in their name, despite much experimentation with citizens' charters. Overall, the last 20 years have seen a shift in the accent of accountability, and hence of audit and monitoring, from an input focus on costs and process to an output focus on the quality of service delivered, a point which will be taken up further below.

A fourth factor, which may be as much effect as cause, is a conspicuous loss of trust in service professionals in the public sector. Variability, non-comparability and idiosyncrasy in practice have become illegitimate for a political system dedicated to a transparent and equitable quality of service. It is argued that clinical judgement combines standard diagnostic templates with a seasoned sensitivity to the particularities of the case. Not only does standardisation mis-characterise the nature of the service, it is also a bad way to organise science (Charlton 1993). However, this line of critique has done little to temper an institutionalised commitment to making professional judgement visible beyond its local settings. Trust has shifted systemically from professionals to auditors, inspectors, evaluators and related management activity.

The abiding irony of these changes is that rhetoric of accountability and transparency can never be fully lived by organisations. The models of organisation and clinical practice embedded in the operating assumptions of NICE and CHI are likely to be highly unrealistic ones, idealisations which must, at great expense, be created almost uniquely for the purpose of being audited and inspected. From this point of view, audit and inspection are not simply a technical means to secure accountability; they also construct organisational realities.

Elements of audit and inspection

Despite the rationality of the programmes which set them in motion (such as the Health Act 1999), monitoring practices which get called audit and inspection are messy and *ad hoc* assemblies of tools and procedures. The Audit Commission (1999) distinguishes between audit and inspection in terms of an emphasis on financial cost and an emphasis on quality of performance, respectively. This is a useful view, but also much too neat. Rather than attempting to elaborate a refined basis for distinguishing audit and inspection, it is much more useful to identify the various elements that may be more or less present in each. This will be helpful in addressing the peculiarities of what has come to be called 'clinical' auditing.

First, an emphasis on financial regularity and legality has a long history and remains an important objective of audit processes, despite being regarded as humble and routine by many practitioners. Second, there has also been a reasonably long history of concern with cost-effectiveness in public sector auditing. Cost-effectiveness is a more elusive concept than it might seem since it relates cost inputs to some kind of auditable performance-based output. Research suggests that in many settings where the effectiveness of public services is ambivalent or difficult to demonstrate (e.g. child care or psychotherapy), cost-effectiveness gravitates to the cheapest option (Power 1998). What is clear and relevant to the case of NICE is that quality and cost-effectiveness relate to different and competing 'logics of evaluation'; it is not necessarily the case that they can be combined seamlessly. Indeed, whether NICE can rebut charges of rationing will depend on precisely how these different logics are combined.

For many years in the UK, regularity and cost-effectiveness were the core objectives of value-for-money auditing in the public sector. However, the 'audit' process was also more of an advisory practice with the goal of reforming organisations in order to embed an operational emphasis on cost-effectiveness. In recent years, and particularly since the change in the UK Government in 1997, the effectiveness dimension of value-for-money auditing, i.e. the quality of services, has become increasingly emphasised. Indeed, there is now widespread commitment to relate quality to outcomes which may be less amenable to observation (e.g. responsible citizens) and not merely to easily measurable outputs (e.g. exam results). In short, the third 'E' of the three E's of value-for-money auditing (Economy, Efficiency and Effectiveness) is playing a greater role in political discourse and policy discussion than ever before.

With this shift in policy emphasis, it is clear that the design of appropriate performance measures and standards is central to audit and inspection activity. NICE will develop the standards that will be audited by CHI. The logic seems simple enough: organisations like NICE will evaluate existing practices and inductively derive standards for excellence which will be disseminated around the system as norms of conduct. CHI will then be in a position to verify compliance with the norms and enact sanctions as required. From this point of view, the development of standards supports and enables the inspection activity. The lynchpin of this entire system is clinical auditing.

Clinical governance, audit and CHI

Regulatory systems rarely emerge out of the blue. Financial regulation has developed as a series of residues left behind by scandals, each new scandal bringing a fresh rewriting of the rules. Similarly, the voluntary code for corporate governance had its origins in a series of reactions to the collapse of the Maxwell empire. It is worth reminding medical practitioners of this historical path since organisations like NICE and CHI tend not to remember their own origins. The unacceptability of variation in clinical judgement (and cost) has emerged partly from ideological commitment and partly from scandal, such as the Bristol case.

Clinical audit is at the centre of the re-invention of clinical governance in the health care system. 'Clinical audit' is perhaps a misleading label, since the concept has a very different origin from that of financial audit and resembles it in name and little more. Clinical audit began as a local and idiosyncratic practice of reflection on clinical results (Exworthy 1999). Indeed, the process was more akin to an assessment or review or even research than to the generally accepted idea of audit as independent verification. However, sometime in the 1980s in the UK, this review activity was termed 'audit'. Once this new label was attached, the practice could be thought about in a new way in relation to the management of health care. It became possible to think of it as a basis for a different kind of intervention in, and control of, clinical practice. And as local and *ad hoc* forms of self-audit decreased in legitimacy, clinical audit started to turn into something which it never used to be, i.e. a vehicle for the independent enforcement of clinical standards. The perceived failure and ideological unacceptability of *ad hoc* self-appraisal systems have meant not only that localism in medical practice is giving way to centralism and standardisation, but also that there is a new de-politicisation of the health care field.

This process of transformation in the status and functioning of clinical audit reaches an important point with the advent of NICE and CHI, organisations committed to realising clinical governance by making medical practice auditable and inspectable. Rawlins (1999) has identified the problems giving rise to the need for NICE: waste, dubious clinical effectiveness, delays in introducing new methods. NICE will be engaged in the appraisal of new techniques, the development of clinical guidelines and the performance of clinical audit. The appraisal activity, which is beyond the scope of this chapter, has an impact on the territory of science and raises issues about the model of science with which NICE will work (see Charlton 1993 and Chapter 2 of this volume) and its authority in relation to the pharmaceutical industry. The writing of guidelines raises further issues about the very possibility of designing judgement out of practice via standards (see Chapter 1 of this volume). Such guidance is not merely about ensuring best practice, but is also required to make practice auditable.

Overall, NICE intends to be a network organisation by harnessing external expertise where necessary and by building multiple alliances with practice and with industry. As an important part of the strategy for 'clinical governance' within health services, it functions as a buffer between the political system and the service delivery system. In this way, typical of inspectorates and audit institutions, it plays a certain kind of role in de-politicising the field, even at the same time as many of its choices in the field of clinical practice will be political as well as medical. The development of standards, which will be monitored by CHI, is the continuation of centralism by other means.

The Commission for Health Improvement

The Commission will directly assist the work of NICE. Indeed, the Secretary of State for Health has made it clear that he expects 'health service organisations systematically and consistently to take account of NICE's guidelines' and that '... the new Commission for Health Improvement will help ensure this happens' (Beecham 2000). Furthermore, Professor Sir Michael Rawlins, Chairman of NICE, when discussing CHI's likely attitude to variations, has confirmed that 'there would be no flexibility – no deviation. CHI would come and the roof would fall in' (Rawlins, quoted in Hutchinson 1999). The Commission derives its inspectorial and advisory function from section 18 of the Health Act 1999. It has wide-ranging powers of information gathering (section 19) subject to various qualifications (most of them lobbied for successfully by the BMA) and has a duty to operate itself with economy, efficiency and effectiveness (meaning that CHI will be audited itself). The announcement is made that CHI will 'eradicate second-rate care' (Dunne 1999a) and begin its work in April 2000 with a mission to:

'... raise the standard of clinical governance across the NHS; a quantum leap in service quality which will make a direct impact on the patient experience. We will be a developmental, facilitative and regulatory independent body.

Where good practice is found, we will spread that knowledge. Where advice is required, we will be able to draw upon experience across the breadth of the NHS ...' (Classifieds 2000).

It must be asked whether CHI is a genuine experiment in quality control which will be sensitive to local operating conditions, or whether it is a tool of central government ideologically committed to central control of professional groups. The answer will not be known for many years, but is likely to be a mixture of both. Much will depend on operational relations between NICE, CHI and other inspectors (e.g. Audit Commission), especially as the coherence of public sector audit and inspection activity has been widely debated. CHI will need to develop its own distinctive operational style, dependent on its direct expertise assets and perceived legitimacy in the health system. Inspectorates can have very different styles of operation, which are only loosely based on their formal powers (Day & Klein 1990).

From an infra-structural standpoint, CHI appointed a chairman and chief executive in late 1999 (Healy 1999) and the 20 January 2000 issue of the *Health Service Journal* (Classifieds 2000) advertises a raft of new executive and impressively remunerated appointments for a director of policy and development, a medical director, a nursing director, a director of information and clinical governance reviews, a director of finance and corporate governance, and a director of communications. From a functional standpoint, the Prime Minister envisages the development of CHI into 'a standards watchdog that will go round every hospital and PCG in the country promoting good practice and high standards and rooting out the bad ... [that] will check that the best treatments as recommended by the National Institute for Clinical Excellence are being used' (McSmith 1999).

A particularly important issue for CHI is the fact that, like any audit or inspection function, its role is highly dependent on the quality of clinical standards issued by NICE. As Loughlin (in Chapter 1 of this volume) shows, all standards require judgement to be applied; hence judgement can never be eliminated. Much will depend on the style of clinical guidelines and whether they are likely to be tightly prescriptive or whether they establish broad principles which allow for local interpretation. Particular standards will vary in style according to the respective states of scientific knowledge and clinical consensus. One can predict that CHI will become more significant than NICE because it will play the key role in determining the legitimacy of interpretative variation in clinical operations and in defining the meaning of compliance itself *in situ* (Hutter 1997).

At its inception in 1999, CHI announced that it intended to review every unit under its remit over the first two years. This is a reasonable strategy for an organisation that must build working alliances with trusts and health authorities, and must establish its operational style and legitimacy within the system. Less realistic may be the more recent announcement of a governmental aspiration for the review of all hospitals and PCGs with a subsequent publication of the results every four years (Donnelly 2000). A reaction from the clinical governance review group of the Commission indicates, however, that CHI will begin its clinical governance review in April 2000 with a pilot study of only acute NHS trusts which 'would not be the worst or the best' in the country but would instead be a 'spread' to test the methodology being developed with a PCG review team to 'follow on behind' the trust programme (Causley, quoted in Donnelly 2000). Some inspectorates, like the National Audit Office, divide their work between routine periodic visits and a rolling programme of special issues (some of which are driven by the political process). Others, like the Audit Commission, are looking to make the routine end of operations more risk-based and more responsive to the self-inspecting capability of organisations. Interestingly, CHI has recently confirmed that it will study the methodologies of the Audit Commission to minimise duplication (Causley, quoted in Donnelly 2000) and a 24-member special advisory group has been constituted to provide strategic guidance on the structure and function of CHI (Dunne 1999b). The advisory group has, however, been criticised for its dramatic under-representation of doctors from routine clinical practice (Dunne 1999b) and concerns remain in relation to how precisely CHI will eventually work with 'other agencies and bodies that presently sit in judgement over NHS organisations ... in particular ... with the Audit Commission, the medical Royal Colleges, the health service ombudsman and the performance management function of regional offices' (Thornton, quoted in McSmith 1999). The question of responsiveness is important for the future of CHI. Given its central position in the system, the scope of operations and its predicted resource base, CHI will operate predominantly in the mode of 'control of control' (Power 1999), that is, at the heart of risk-based approaches. The primary focus will be upon local clinical governance systems for ensuring and monitoring quality and the new National Service Frameworks are likely to play an important role in this context (Chapman 1999). Poor systems and control weaknesses act as a first-level trigger for deeper and more detailed inspection. Equally, a good track record of clinical governance can be rewarded with a light inspectorial touch.

If this risk-based approach is to be realised, it requires a distinctive balance between the classical roles of policeman and consultant. Both roles are possible but they bite at different stages of the inspection process. Borrowing from Ayres & Braithwaite's model (1992) of the 'enforcement ladder', inspection routinely operates consensually with a high degree of co-operation and flow of information and advice. From this point of view CHI can fulfil the desired role of adviser and partner in the clinical governance process. However, where control weaknesses or other problems present themselves, CHI has the legal and institutional option to escalate the inspection process, which will become more adversarial as it moves up the 'ladder'. What is important is not the polarised choice between policeman and consultant, but the design of a rich ladder of enforcement opportunities that enable a smooth process of escalation, e.g. from warnings and requirements for system improvements up to the ultimate sanction of revocation of licence and closure.

These questions of regulatory design for CHI also depend on the quality of information that is available to inspectors. While a great deal of routine information may be communicated to it, experience in other sectors suggests that the ability to acquire and process gossip and dirty data is also essential for successful enforcement.

Standards-based clinical audit: micro-level pathologies?

The questions raised above concern the design of CHI. Its potential operational style can be framed as the problem of aligning the incentives of the regulated and the regulator. The ideal is that organisations can be given incentives for self-government and that the inspection regime can operate with a light touch, even as an adviser in a mutual learning process. The problem is that, at the micro-level, organisational reality does not often operate in this way. A number of side-effects and pathologies of the inspection process must be considered.

It must be assumed that there will be considerable impact on climates of professional judgement. The emergence of a 'contractualist' mentality among medical practitioners may be accelerated by the attempts by NICE and CHI to control clinical decision-making. The phenomenon of creative compliance, i.e. complying with the letter but not the spirit of guidance, is well known in accountancy (McBarnet & Whelan 1991) and may surface in medicine as the need to present 'good' clinical practice to the out-side world increases. Demands for transparency and accountability know no end and practitioners will be drawn increasingly into a world of clinical compliance in which tacit knowledge and local trust no longer have legitimacy.

CHI will no doubt stimulate the growth of (costly) medical 'accountancy', and the 'writing-up' of health care decisions for inspection purposes risks becoming as important as treating patients. The importance of representing treatment for official purposes may lead to defensive and risk-averse strategies. It was reported in 1999 that some surgeons were refusing high-risk patients because of concerns for the impact on their reported mortality rates. Such perverse-incentive effects have also been experienced in other sectors.

Another possible side-effect of the risk-based approach discussed above is a tendency to focus on systems of clinical governance and not on the quality of real treatment. As new experts in clinical audit begin to populate health organisations, the systems which CHI will wish to inspect can become worlds unto themselves, created and maintained to present an inspectable face to the outside world. Perfectly documented procedures, clear flowcharts linking objectives to performance, tightly defined roles, clinical governance manuals for staff and other forms of representation can blind an inspector to what is really going on.

Finally, an important dimension of these side-effects is cost. It is inevitable that compliance costs will increase under NICE and CHI. The economic issues are not simply those of rationing (see Chapter 7 of this volume) but of the cost of creating and running the infrastructure of clinical governance. Compliance costs are difficult to relate to benefits. Furthermore, given the ideological momentum behind NICE, CHI and clinical governance, costs of compliance are more likely to be hidden from view or perceived as resistance and complaining. It can also be predicted that the new regime will give existing clinical auditors an incentive to organise themselves as high-fee advisers to former colleagues and health organisations about how to comply with NICE and CHI. A new industry of compliance consultants will emerge in the shadow of CHI.

Conclusions: CHI and the prospects for 'reflexive inspection'

It is difficult to disagree with the stated objectives of NICE and CHI. They are part of the mood of the times and at the present time we barely have any concepts at all with which to resist greater demands for accountability. Counter-arguments can only be based on empirical evidence, such as the costs relative to benefit and perverse side-effects, but even this assumes a policy process which is amenable to empirical argument of this kind. Bureaucracies tend not to process information that could undermine their own existence.

NICE and CHI have two important constituencies. On the one hand, they act on behalf of, and in the name of, patients. On the other hand, they are also instruments of the political process. In this respect, like other audit and inspection organisations, they function as 'buffers' between the health care system and the political system; they are part of the way the problems get conceptualised and solved for consumption by politics. This systemic role as part of the politics of control is under-analysed, but inspection organisations can be very successful in managerialising issues that might previously have been regarded as political. As more is required of health care organisations in the name of better governance, the state assumes the role of regulator of last resort.

In all this the worst-case scenario is that audit and inspection do not merely have the side-effects described above; they operate almost as a 'fatal remedy' (Sieber 1981). Audit systems and extensive chains of control connecting hospitals to CHI may even function as a 'cover-up' of real issues. This is not a question of individual conspiracy; it is simply that the sheer density of governance structures deflects managerial and political attention from fundamental issues. Control becomes an organisational alibi from other ways of knowing and improving practice. To take the point even further, we face the danger of becoming trapped by our own hyperbole, unable to perceive the real mediocrity beneath the ever-present language of 'excellence'. Organisations have to find ways to ask constantly whether the focus on 'best practice' is beneficial. Is all this highly exacerbated form of performance talk simply the language of decline in disguise?

These issues go far beyond the particular case of CHI, but they are directly relevant to it. From the perspective of 1999, there is an opportunity for the newly created CHI to address and overcome some of these problems and pathologies. Not all these difficulties are under its control and there is a resource constraint. However, the question with which this chapter concludes is whether CHI could be a 'reflexive' inspectorate. This means that it will need to design into itself empirical sensitivity of some kind to side-effects, especially on the incentives of health professionals.

This will not be easy because a bureaucratic style of operation fits uneasily with a style capable of processing diverse information sets. However, CHI is legally required to demonstrate its own effectiveness, presumably in terms of outcomes for better health care. Whether it has the managerial will and ability to process compliance costs and other side-effects remains to be seen; very few organisations close themselves on the grounds that their costs outweigh their benefits.

Much will depend on the concrete operational style adopted by CHI and how it balances its role as consultant and inspector and provides incentives for self-organisation. Lessons can be learned from outside the health arena, such as corporate governance and the recently published Turnbull report (ICAEW 1999) on internal control. Sensitivity to over-monitoring and 'audit exhaustion' will be as important as making an example of failing practice. In all this the credibility of the individual inspectors will be crucial. Monitoring is never neutral, never a mere observation of practice; it is always both relationship-building and the construction of practice itself. As CHI begins its recruitment process, it may face the paradox that it really needs the individuals who would never apply for a position within it.

References

Audit Commission (1998). *Developing principles for public inspection: a consultation document.* The Audit Commission, London.

Ayres I & Braithwaite J (1992). *Responsive regulation: transcending the deregulation debate.* Oxford University Press, Oxford.

Beecham L (2000). Health Secretary sets out NICE's programme. *BMJ* **320**, 63.

Bowerman M, Raby H & Humphrey C (2000). In search of the audit society: some evidence from health care, police and schools. *International Journal of Auditing* **4** (in press).

Chapman G (1999). Developing and delivering National Service Frameworks. *Chief Medical Officer's Update* **23**, 2.

Charlton BG (1993). Management of science. *The Lancet* **342**, 99–100.

Charlton BG (1999). The ideology of 'accountability'. *Journal of the Royal College of Physicians of London* **33**, 33–5.

Classifieds (2000). Lead 'the boldest step yet' in the government's programme to modernise the NHS. *Health Service Journal* 20 Jan, p.57.

Day P & Klein R (1990). *Inspecting the inspectorates.* Joseph Rowntree Foundation, York.

Donnelly L (2000). CHI to pick four sites for reviews. *Health Service Journal* 20 Jan, p.10.

Dunne R (1999a). CHI vows to eradicate 'second-rate' care. *Hospital Doctor* 4 Nov, p.5.

Dunne R (1999b). CHI sets out plan for quality checks. *Hospital Doctor* 2 Sept.

Exworthy M (1998). Clinical audit in the NHS internal market: from peer review to external monitoring. *Public Policy and Administration* **13**, 40–53.

Healy P (1999). On the critical list. *Health Service Journal* 26 Aug, pp.10–11.

Hood C (1991). A public management for all seasons? *Public Administration* **69**, 3–19.

Horton R (1999). NICE: a step forward in the quality of NHS care. *The Lancet* **353**, 1028–9.

Hutchinson M (1999). NICE guy talks tough to win consultants' trust. *Hospital Doctor* 8 Apr, pp.32–3.

Hutter B (1997). *Compliance: regulation and environment.* Oxford University Press, Oxford.

[ICAEW] Institute of Chartered Accountants in England and Wales (1999). *Internal control: guidance for the directors of listed companies incorporated in the United Kingdom.* ICAEW, London.

McBarnet D & Whelan C (1991). The elusive spirit of the law: formalism and the struggle for legal control. *The Modern Law Review* **54**, 874–88.

McSmith A (1999). Prime Minister launches NHS inspectorate. *BMJ* **319**, 1217.

Power M (1994). *The audit explosion.* Demos, London.

Power M (1998). The audit fixation: some issues for psychotherapy. In *Rethinking clinical audit: the case of psychotherapy services in the NHS* (ed. R Davenhill & M Patrick), pp. 23–37. Routledge, London.

Power M (1999). *The audit society: rituals of verification.* Oxford University Press, Oxford.

Rawlins M (1999). In pursuit of quality: the National Institute for Clinical Excellence. *The Lancet* **353**, 1079–82.

Sieber S D (1981). *Fatal remedies: the ironies of social intervention.* Plenum Press, New York, USA.

Smith R (1999). NICE: a panacea for the NHS? *BMJ* **318**, 823–4.

Chapter 10

Analysis by CHI of divergence from NICE-approved guidelines: how will a judgement be made between sub-optimal care and good decision skill?

Philip D Welsby

Introduction

In the preceding chapter, Power describes the statutory powers of the Commission for Health Improvement (CHI) and how, through a variety of developed methodologies and inter-relationships with other regulatory and inspectorial bodies, it will directly assist the implementation of clinical practice guidelines either developed by or approved through the National Institute for Clinical Excellence (NICE). Since the assumed authority of NICE is so great and the statutory powers of CHI so substantial (see particularly Chapters 2, 3 and 9 of this volume), practising clinicians are likely to experience considerable pressures to align their local clinical practice with the directions of nationally promulgated guidelines.

Many clinicians will continue to tailor clinical care to the individual patient, and this is likely to result in divergences from NICE-developed/approved guidelines. Clinical governance is likely to ensure that local information systems are sufficiently developed to come to detect such variations more sensitively, and digests of such internal information will thus become available for external inspection by CHI. In some cases, such divergences will be perfectly justified on clinical grounds. In others, such divergences may be unjustifiable clinically. How, then, will local and national mechanisms of monitoring and inspection make a judgement between good decision skills and sub-optimal care in this context? The present chapter will consider this pivotal matter following an initial discussion of the nature of the complexity in clinical practice.

Clinical practice

There is an epidemic of guidelines, every specialist society has some. To be clear at the start: *no one doubt should that knowledge of guidelines is very important.* Guidelines are important for patient care and for education of the medical profession. But problems arise when their importance is overemphasised. In the past, therapeutic interventions for serious diseases were limited: outcome assessment, identification of their causes, and effects of therapy upon causes were simple and, accordingly, guidelines were simple, with little need to consider how different guidelines might interact. Patients now survive with several co-existing serious conditions such that multiple, interacting guidelines may apply. For example, it is not uncommon for a large proportion of patients, particularly the elderly, to have (say) up to five conditions and in consequence to be receiving (say) up to nine therapies providing 120 potential combinations of underlying diagnoses and at least 362,880 potential combinations of therapies. Although individual patients could each only have a maximum of five interacting guidelines, there is ample opportunity for guideline interactions. Indeed, it would be remarkable if no interactions occurred.

Guidelines, to be educational, should provide reasons for the recommendations. This may be tedious and often the equivalent of a textbook. For example, in one set of meningitis guidelines 'a consensus statement' consists of 11,252 words (Begg *et al.* 1999). The alternative would be briefer, but unacceptable, *ex cathedra* guidelines.

Written guidelines often deal with *diagnoses* and are restricted to one dimension, quite literally, reading left to right. Guidelines are often presented as flowcharts (Figure 10.1) in two dimensions (left to right and up and down). However, *patients* and their clinicians function in a four-dimensional world, and flowcharts, if they are to reflect reality, should also be four-dimensional (i.e. left to right, up and down, front and back, and altering with time).

In the Infectious Diseases Unit in which I work regular audits are performed in which practice is compared against guidelines. Often some aspect of the management of various patients differs from accepted guidelines. In nearly all patients there might have been very good reasons for non-guideline treatments arising from factors that were not (and could not reasonably be expected to be) covered by the guidelines for treatment of individual conditions. So what was the function of these guidelines? They made us question our practice. They made us think.

Figure 10.1 shows an archetypal guideline for a condition in which symptoms and signs lead to a definite diagnosis from which therapy follows *if, and only if, symptoms and signs elicited are precise and a single definite diagnosis can be reached* ('Type I complexity'). Simple problem orientation flows in towards a diagnosis and simple guidelines flow out – a triumph of reductionism, which works for simple conditions. The archetypal simple single condition is, of course, sudden death and no one would question that guidelines for resuscitation are appropriate and adherence to such guidelines could be used to assess competence of care.

However, patients often have several diagnoses and superimposition of, say, five Figure 10.1 guidelines results in a literally mind-boggling 'Type II complexity' (Figure 10.2). This is bad enough but most clinicians who do post-take ward rounds find that the initial task is not the establishment of diagnoses and treatment utilising 'Type I complexity' guidelines but rather deciding what should be done while

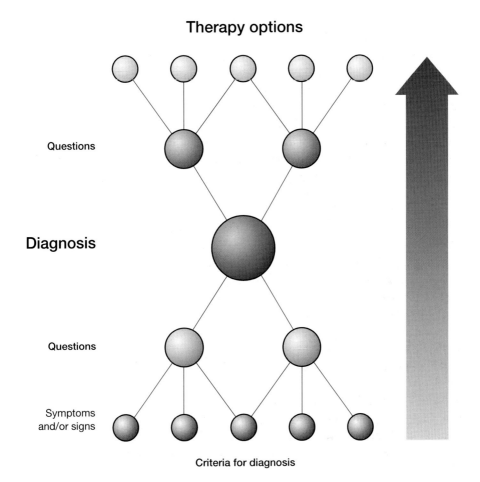

Figure 10.1 Type I complexity

diagnoses are being established. If symptoms and signs are equivocal, there will be diagnostic doubt. In fact, there are 29 official gradings of uncertainty and only one of certainty (Beyth-Maron 1982)!

In such patients there may be a mass of *pre-diagnostic* intertwining management possibilities (for which there are no written guidelines), and the branches leading to and from the diagnostic stem will therefore be blurred. Worse, the diagnoses or treatments may interact with each other resulting in the maze of 'Type III complexity' (Figure 10.3). Guidelines are often derived from controlled trials of simplified situations using criteria that often exclude other complicating serious conditions. Thus simple 'Type I complexity' guidelines may not be applicable to complex situations (see Chapter 3 of this volume).

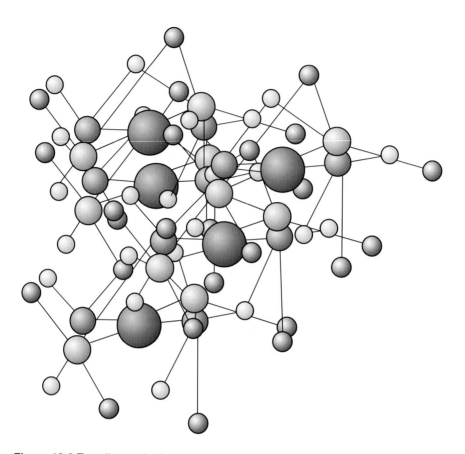

Figure 10.2 Type II complexity

Medical information is often statistical ('we are 75 per cent certain that ...') and is basically analogue (positive merging into negative) rather than digital (yes or no). Guidelines are essentially digital. To round off analogue information into digital form is to run the risk that you pay in accuracy and honesty for what you gain in simplicity.

Somewhere, hidden in these complex interacting guidelines, is the art of medicine and, as in life in general, important decisions have to be made using incomplete information (in infectious diseases, my specialty, this is almost always the case and diagnoses are often confirmed only after therapy has been given). Currently undervalued attributes like clinical experience become important.

There are two ways to deal with Type II and III complexity. Some clinicians, the reductionist tacticians, when presented with Type II and III complexity, approach the complexity maze bearing volumes of rigid guidelines and try to analyse all possible routes, thus spending a lot of time in discussion before coming to any decision. I suspect

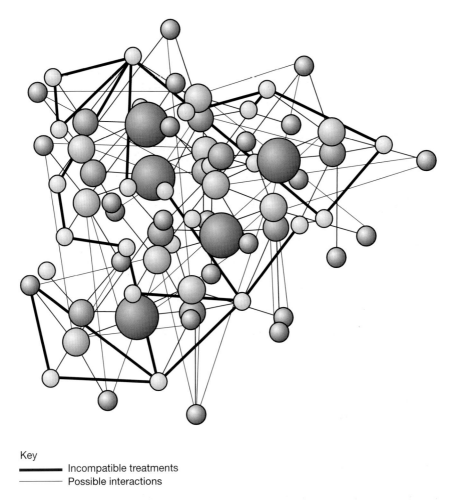

Key

━━━━━━━ Incompatible treatments
─────── Possible interactions

Figure 10.3 Type III complexity

it will be easy to demonstrate at least one instance of poor practice as judged by failure to adhere to a guideline *in retrospect* (even where the outcomes are satisfactory), but when confronted with Type II or III complexity *in prospect,* it will often be difficult to say what is the best route through the maze. Other clinicians, the strategists, metaphorically float above the situation and abstract what seems to be the best plan of action (it is easier to get through a maze if you can take an overview) and avoid crossing the maze by asking questions along the lines of 'What would happen if we did X?'; but it seems that few clinicians have minds that can mechanically analyse and float simultaneously. It would be ideal for doctors to achieve a balance using both methods. If management of complex patients could be reduced to guidelines and were wholly algorithmic, then we should all start programming computers with such guidelines and then retire. If guidelines for specific conditions are applicable, do we need a doctor's skill to apply them after the diagnosis has been made?

In the clinical unit in which I work I used to be unhappy about disagreements about the management of certain complex patients with HIV disease until I realised that individual colleagues were each entering the complexity maze by different routes (Figure 10.4), while bearing the same guidelines which they interpreted from different viewpoints. This is an example of how the stress on local ownership of guidelines can mean individual ownership, which does lessen their value.

Assessment of clinical competence

The foundational principle for the creation and institution of NICE and CHI is that of increasing quality in the NHS by a 'quantum leap'. Theoretically, at least, NICE will promulgate clinical practice guidelines that incorporate the latest knowledge and reflect the latest health policies, and compliance with them is an explicit expectation of both institutions. Divergence from these national guidelines may come to be common place as good clinicians seek to tailor care to individual patients. The assessment of 'clinical competence' may in part involve an assessment of the number and appropriateness of divergences from these national guidelines in order to differentiate 'good' from 'bad' clinical practice in the context of the individual clinical case.

So how will a judgement be made between sub-optimal care and good decision skill? For simple single conditions assessment of adherence to an agreed guideline would seem an appropriate initial way to ensure quality of health care. No one would question that the adherence to resuscitation guidelines can be used as a measure of care in the ultimate simple situation, cardiorespiratory arrest. However, with complex patients adherence to multiple guidelines may not be an appropriate measure of quality of care.

How then should competence be assessed? With complex patients the clinical outcome would seem to be the most important judge of quality of care. But the use of outcome league tables to identify poorly performing units worthy of CHI attention is fallible. Poor results can be caused by case-mix fluctuations or by chance. Identification of case-mix fluctuations requires well-validated adjustment models and resources to collect data. However, if units treat less than several hundred patients with simple, single, easily defined conditions, then the role of chance will be such that the majority of units in the bottom, say, 20 per cent of an outcome league table will probably not be performing poorly. Nevertheless, they will have been identified as performing poorly and could be investigated by CHI, who will almost inevitably find a failure to adhere fully to at least one guideline from all possible applicable guidelines in complex patients. If most units at the bottom of the league table are actually average or good performers who have been unlucky, then the chances are that their results will be better subsequently (they will regress to the mean) and *any* intervention will be perceived to have succeeded. The risks of the uncritical utilisation of performance indicators have been succinctly reviewed by Signorini (1999) (Figure 10.5).

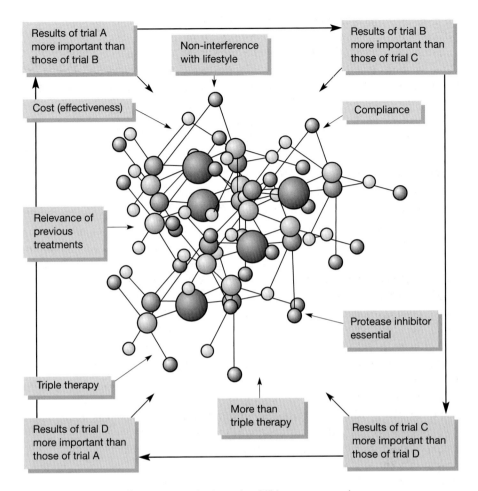

Figure 10.4 Approaches to complexity using HIV as an example

The CHI 'hit squads', if we may use a pejorative term to describe the new inspectorate, will succeed for much the same reason that stock market traders purchase good shares that by chance happen to be poorly performing: 'buy-low' and then just wait for them to improve: 'sell-high.' CHI squads will also succeed because they will have the luxury of making judgements in retrospect. The assessment of reasons underlying poor outcomes will thus be complex and controversial. Additionally, clinicians under study will alter their practice. In New York the publication of performance reports resulted in a 'questionable' reduction in operative mortality because surgeons were reluctant to operate on higher risk patients (Green & Wintfeld 1995; Schneider & Epstein 1996).

Before I learned that one major function of CHI was to audit against NICE guidelines to evaluate and monitor clinical practice, I was only mildly uneasy about what I perceived to be increasing reductionism in medicine and thought that, on balance, it

Key
Upper case = objective occurrences
Lower case = uninformed opinion

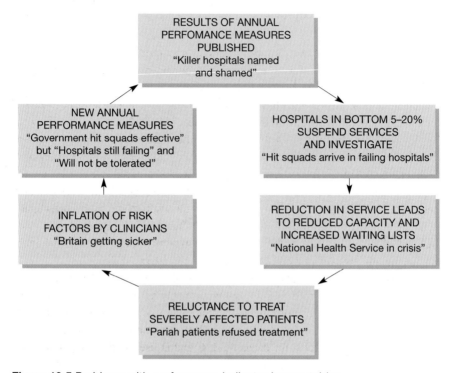

Figure 10.5 Problems with performance indicator league tables

might be helpful; however, I now believe that the intention to use guidelines reveals reductionism to be running wild. It is inappropriate and unbalanced, and it ignores Type II and III complexity. If it is allowed to succeed, those of us who deal with Type II and III complexity will be spending most of our time explaining why there were special circumstances that applied to particular patients even if our performance indicators were good. It could be argued that we have to accept that 'we have to be accountable', but I suspect more of those with generalist leanings will in future opt for a quieter life by entering reductionist specialties. I have no argument against reductionism in general. Indeed reductionism, by focusing on particular questions, has been a major method of scientific discovery but I am against the idea that the quality of care of complex patients merely comprises the serial ascertainment of fixed, non-interactive diagnoses that will yield to serial application of Type I complexity guidelines. The medical profession recognises this when things go wrong and guidelines do not work, as they do from time to time, when we say that the patient has 'developed complications.' Patients do not develop complications, but rather reveal previously unsuspected complexity.

Evidence-based medicine: the foundation of guidelines

Evidence-based medicine (EBM) is the conscious, explicit and judicious use of current best evidence in making decisions about the care of individual patients (Sackett *et al.* 1996). EBM can answer the question, 'What is the best treatment for *condition X?*', but for *patients* with Type II and III complexity there may often, or perhaps almost always, be no single EBM answer available. Using sequences of Type I complexity guidelines through Type II and III complexity may produce a pathway through the maze which, although incontrovertible, *may not be the best pathway.* Even the sequence in which guidelines are implemented may influence the result.

Clinical trials are usually the basis of EBM. Obviously, statistical results obtained from trials are generalisations that may not apply to individuals. However, generalisations (the old, well-established idea for the new concept of statistical analysis) are now so highly sophisticated that errors are usually made at a fundamental level by acceptance of assumptions that are so basic that they are usually ignored. Results of studies conducted in one place at one time are assumed to be applicable in other places at other times. With HIV, for example, we assume that results from one trial in one country at one time, in different racial groups, with different genetic backgrounds, with different (often ongoing) at-risk behaviours, are universally applicable, even when the virus continually mutates and resistance patterns will differ.

I have one slight worry about meta-analysis as a tool for assembling EBM guidelines. Drawing conclusions from sequences of several trials of therapies, each of which producing results showing that one therapy is better than another, may be inappropriate if the sequence is non-transitive. Figure 10.6 illustrates non-transitivity. If, say, dice A, B, C and D are substituted for drugs A, B, C and D used in three separate trials, drug A versus drug B, drug B versus drug C, and drug C versus drug D, and each drug has six numerically graded parameters (e.g. clinical action, bioavailability, absorption, excretion, side-effects, metabolism) as the numbers on the dice, then there is a sequence in which A is better that B, B is better than C, C is better than D but *almost* unbelievably D is better than A! This counter-intuitive finding was first noted by Efron (1990). I do not know how common such non-transitivity might be in drug trials but there are numerous recommendations based on drug A being better than drug B in one trial, drug B being better than drug C in another trial, which in another trial, is better than drug D. Can it be necessarily concluded that drug A is the best drug?

Which of us runs an evidence-based life, anyway? Which of us performed a prospective double-blind randomised controlled trial to evaluate our future spouse? Do we all obey the Consumers Association *Which?* reports?

In spite of all the above reflections there can be little doubt that medicine based on best evidence is preferable despite the reservations expressed in the *Journal of Clinical Evaluation* thematic issue on medical education (Norman 1999) and despite the fact that some medical schools accept alternative medicine into their curricula despite the lack of scientific basis for most complementary therapies.

Problem-oriented medical records

Reductionism has been tried before in the shape of 'problem-oriented medical records' and did not achieve popular acceptance. Problem-oriented medical records reduced a patient's totality to a list of problems, each of which was addressed in turn. Why did they not succeed? I suspect the main reason was that most clinicians intuitively realised that such Type I processing of patients did not address, indeed may have impaired, overall management of Type II and III complexity by forcing patients' complaints through a reductionist problem sieve.

It may be more relevant to ask the question, 'What is going on here in this patient?' and provide an integrated answer rather than attempting to enumerate the isolated problems.

The human mind

Why is reductionism popular? Probably because it is one way in which the *conscious* human mind attempts to cope with Type II and III complexity. Unfortunately, the human mind cannot adequately deal with such complexities because they overwhelm the brain's random access memory and processing power. In particular, the human mind cannot cope with *simultaneous* parallel processing and integration of Type II and III complexity. This simultaneity is important because the mathematics of matrixes reveals that the order in which interrelated problems are addressed may affect the outcome (put simply, if you blindly select two socks from a drawer in which there are two blue socks and one red sock, you will stand a 50 per cent chance of obtaining a pair if you first pick a blue sock, but no chance if you first pick a red sock). Dealing with

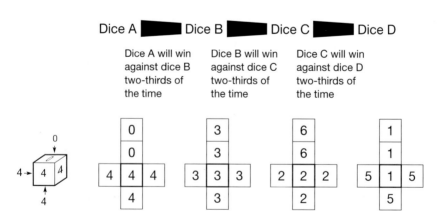

Dice D will win against dice A two-thirds of the time

Figure 10.6 Non-transitivity

an integrated set of problems as if each problem were capable of solution in isolation and could be addressed sequentially is not likely to reveal integrated solutions.

It is true that some geniuses can cope with multifaceted complexity – Mozart produced much of his music from his *unconscious* mind without knowing how. The rest of us need to accept the inadequacies of our minds. That human consciousness cannot deal with Type II complexity is not an excuse to abandon unscientific thought in favour of mysticism (although it does explain why mysticism attracts the woolly minded).

I believe that ultimately computers will triumph in many complex situations as well as they do in chess because they will be able to assess all possible guideline-derived pathways in all sequences through Type II and III complexity. However, with each additional diagnosis the amount of computer space and time required for solutions increases exponentially. The fact remains that the computer input will have to be performed by clinicians who will have to interpret patients' complaints into computer form.

Computers are better at dealing with Type II and III complexity precisely because we are human. It is reported that Kasparov lost to the chess computer Deep Blue (a *strictly* guideline-driven machine playing a rigidly defined game) not because he was an inferior chess player but because he was ground down by the constant battle (each time he moved a chess piece after much thought the computer replied almost instantly giving his brain no time in which to recover function in human fashion). Clinicians play on a board of uncertain size, with squares of uncertain size, with pieces (of information) that are fuzzy, and in which movements of one piece may affect other pieces.

The future is awaited with interest, but I doubt if an assumption that humans have the mind power to compete with computers is the way forward.

Some implications for medical education

Guidelines, predictably, are usually written by self-selected groups of high achievers who are at or near the top of their career pyramid. They tend to be focused, analytical, self-confident, ambitious, militantly enthusiastic and highly intelligent specialists (usually professors). The members of such groups tend to have precise, box-like memories such that they can rapidly construct Type I complexity guidelines. These distinctly unusual groupings tend to be led by those who have a major influence on teaching programmes. I fear we run the risk that such leaders are leading us to an increase in reductionism. Appreciation of the 'big picture,' surely a fundamental aim of medical education, will not be achieved by trotting out a succession of reductionist 'little picture' guidelines. The most balanced view of Type II and III complexity might well be from a non-reductionist, relatively unfocused general clinician. I repeat: this is not decrying guidelines. *No one doubt should that knowledge of guidelines is very important* (especially for single simple problems).

It seems there has to be a hope that knowledge of guidelines will compensate for lack of clinical experience. Consultants are now appointed at an average age of 33 (previously 35–40), have now been trained using one-in-five rotas (previously one in three), with 72 hours worked each week, and the number of hours' experience before consultant appointments is now 12,880 (previously 25,760). Doctors are thus being produced who have great clinical experience of guidelines and protocols (but not of individual patients and this is by any standards alarming).

General clinical services, teaching and research (researchers are almost invariably specialists and, sadly, specialisation implies reductionism) are three different but complementary activities. However, research depends in large part on reductionism. Thus the assumption that research 'the University approach' offers the best balance for education of those who will provide general clinical services may not be correct. We presently have a pattern that future clinicians may spend years chasing lymphocytes and rats to enhance their chance of a clinical post. Providing a minor change in emphasis with increased generalist teaching by clinicians who are service providers may suffice to correct the imbalance. For example, lectures by specialists could be attended by an appropriate generalist clinician who could be given ten minutes at the end to put the presentation in context. Students could then be advised as to what they need to retain as core knowledge, what should be regarded as background knowledge, and what they do not need to know. Enthusiastic researchers or specialists would not betray their enthusiasm or specialty thus!

A hypothesis cannot stand if one of its foundations can be shown to be false. The current covert hypothesis seems to be that medical training is unbalanced and needs to be corrected by increasing reductionism (including the introduction of Type I guidelines). This hypothesis must have, as a foundation, that an unbalanced number of students are currently favouring 'holistic complexity appreciation practice' rather than reductionism. But junior doctors are doing the reverse and favouring specialist practice rather than general practice. The hypothesis fails. Medical students and doctors in training should experience the various ways in which various clinicians handle Type II and III complexity, not just how they handle Type I guidelines.

There is a reductionist assumption that all would be well if we all were to exchange guidelines. We should encourage the insight that Type II and III complexity exists and is important. I have suggested a 'new' concept for a well-established old idea – a paradigm shift to patient- (rather than condition-) led, experience-based medicine (sounds impressive, does it not?) by increasing the input from generalist clinicians who can put things in complexity context and who would put the general before the particular to allow students to accumulate complexity management within their own framework (Welsby 1999). Put simply, we ought to revalue the role of clinical experience and educational programmes, and journals should address the inevitable complexity associated with modern patients.

If we retain, as I think we should, medical courses that try to produce 'well-rounded, general purpose doctors,' and do not aim for specialism at the start – eschewing 'a surgical, or medical, or radiological, or microbiological medical student' – then we need to address the problem of how to manage *whole patients* in whom multi-system, multi-specialty, multi-guideline conditions appertain.

Guidelines – a marketing disaster?

There is a major fear, which may or may not be justified, that CHI or the legal profession might use NICE guidelines to enforce their wishes upon us. Guidelines often seem to evoke strong negative reactions. There are, I think, two reasons for this.

First, the term 'guidelines' contains the word 'lines', which has unfortunate, quasi-military associations (e.g. 'lines have been drawn up'). Lines are drawn by rulers, tend to be inflexible, are often used to box things in and scientifically have length but no breadth. These associations offend the exquisite sensitivity of doctors. Professor Sir Michael Rawlins, the chairman of NICE, appears regularly in the media to rebut the rich flow of medical paranoia which is cannulated each time the word 'guideline' is mentioned. My advice would be for NICE to rename their recommendations 'guidance' and then market them with a militantly constructive attitude. At least one set of guidelines was termed 'a consensus statement' to avoid provoking unnecessary reactions (Begg *et al.* 1999).

Second, the proposed use of guidelines ignores human nature. People who think, rightly or wrongly, that they are doing their best do not respond positively to criticism, whether it be real or perceived. They respond to advice and help. Alienating the workforce may not matter if the workforce is performing simple tasks under supervision, but if the workforce is performing complex tasks unsupervised, then there will be problems.

Conclusions

Guidelines are useful for simple single conditions and adherence to agreed guidelines could be used as an initial assessment of quality of care. The problem is patients and their complexity. The hope that simple approaches, such as auditing, compliance with guidelines and performance indicators, can be used to assess clinical care of complex situations is over-optimistic. Guidelines should be renamed 'guidance' to avoid the fear that, despite the avowal of their developers, the guidelines could be used to impose inappropriate constraints on medical practice.

References

Begg N *et al.* (1999). British Infection Society consensus statement on diagnosis, investigation, treatment and prevention of acute bacterial meningitis in immunocompetent adults. *Journal of Infection* **39**, 1–15.

Beyth-Maron R (1982). How probable is probable? *Journal of Forecasting* **1**, 257–69.

Efron B (1990). Described in Paulos JA *Innumeracy*. Penguin Books, Harmondsworth, p.100.

Green J & Wintfeld N. Report cards on cardiac surgeons. *N Engl J Med* **332**, 1229–32.

Norman GR (1999). Examining the assumptions of evidence-based medicine. *Journal of Evaluation in Clinical Practice* **5**, 139–47.

Sackett D, Richardson WS, Rosenberg W & Haynes P (1996). *Evidence-based medicine.* Churchill Livingstone, London.

Schneider EC & Epstein AM (1996). Influence of cardiac surgery performance reports on referral practices and access to care. *N Engl J Med* **335**, 251–6.

Signorini DE (1999). League tables: useful tool or dangerous misinformation. *Chiron* (Newsletter of the Royal College of Physicians of Edinburgh) May, 8.

Welsby PD (1999). Reductionism in medicine: some thoughts on medical education from the clinical front line. *Journal of Evaluation in Clinical Practice* **5**, 125–31.

Chapter 11

Clinical guidelines, NICE products and legal liability?

Brian Hurwitz

> *'Guidelines have no defined legal position. However, any doctor not fulfilling the standards and quality of care in the appropriate treatment that are set out in these Clinical Guidelines, will have this taken into account if, for any reason, consideration of their performance in this clinical area is undertaken.'*
>
> (Department of Health 1999a, p.xv)

Introduction

Development of clinical guidelines in the UK has hitherto been undertaken by many organisations, including the Department of Health (DoH), medical Royal Colleges, specialist associations, purchasing authorities, hospital providers, patient groups, and alliances of these organisations (Hurwitz 1998). Despite concerns over variability of guideline advice (Sudlow & Thomson 1997; Thomson *et al.* 1998) and complaints by clinicians of 'guideline overload and fatigue', their use has now been further endorsed by the General Medical Council (1998, p.8), which has announced that 'clinical teams will normally use recommended clinical guidelines'.

As guidelines receive increasing acceptance in the clinical community, health service lawyers have argued that acting in accordance with them could come to be viewed as acceptable medical practice *per se* (Stern 1995; Montgomery 1997) and conversely, therefore, failure to apply a guideline could result in clinicians having a *prima facie* case to answer.

Definitions

A widely adopted definition developed by the US Institute of Medicine views clinical guidelines as 'systematically developed statements to assist practitioner and patient decisions about appropriate health care for specific clinical circumstances' (Field & Lohr 1990, p.8). This encapsulation has gained acceptance in the UK too, but it offers little indication of the standard-setting potential or the regulatory role now accorded to clinical guidelines, and it leaves untheorised the interrelationship between guidelines and their users.

Wider context

Rigid, uncritical adherence to guidelines has not so far been the formal, administrative or managerial expectation in the NHS. But just how widespread is the interest in the potential regulatory role of guidelines is evidenced by a dialogue (quoted in Norton-Taylor 1995, p.239) that took place in the 1996 Scott Inquiry (Scott 1996) – a judicial inquiry which considered whether four guidelines concerning the sale of arms to Iran and Iraq had, or had not, been broken by the Thatcher Government:[1]

Lawyer   Some of the witnesses we have had have described these guidelines as a framework, within which to work ... Does that fit in with how you saw the guidelines?

Lady Thatcher: They are exactly what they say, guidelines, they are not the law. They are guidelines.

Lawyer: Did they have to be followed?

Lady Thatcher: Of course they have to be followed, but they are not strict law. That is why they are guidelines and not law and, of course, they have to be applied according to the relevant circumstances.

Lawyer: Are they expected to be followed?

Lady Thatcher: Of course they have to be followed. They need to be followed for what they are, guidelines.

This exchange vividly demonstrates the appeal of guidelines to authorities attempting to enforce accountability. If documents labelled 'guidelines' can properly evoke expectations that their recommendations be adhered to, even by prime ministers, do they not place clinicians under legal obligations too?

The NHS Executive (1996, p.10) has stated that, when endorsed by prestigious professional bodies, 'clinical guidelines can still only assist the practitioner; they cannot be used to mandate, authorise or outlaw treatment options. Regardless of the strength of the evidence, it will remain the responsibility of the practising clinicians to interpret their application ... It would be wholly inappropriate for clinical guidelines to be used as a means of coercion of the individual clinician'.

---

1   This report, which took three years to compile, ran to over a million words in its consideration of whether four guidelines, expressed in a mere 80 words, concerning the sale of arms to Iran and Iraq, had or had not been breached. The guidelines were originally drawn up by officials from the Foreign Office and the Ministry of Defence, and also concerned the Department of Trade and Industry. Each government department apparently had its own view about the degree of flexibility permitted by the guidelines.

Minimum standard of medical care

The legally required standard of medical care that a doctor owes a patient derives in the UK from the case of *Bolam* v *Friern Hospital Management Committee* (1957). Doctors can successfully defend a charge of negligence if they can show that they have acted in a manner judged appropriate by a body of other responsible doctors. In the words of the judge of this case, 'the test is the standard of the ordinary skilled man exercising and professing to have that special skill'. Expert testimony helps the courts to ascertain what is accepted and proper practice in specific cases, and this generally ensures that professionally generated standards – so called *customary* standards – are applied in the UK rather than standards from elsewhere (e.g. from clinical guidelines) (Lord Scarman 1987, p.132).

Although UK courts have taken note of guidelines (*Re F* 1989; *In re A and others* 1991), they have not so far credited guidelines with a special legal value. But, arguably, such legal cases as have occurred were heard in a previous era, when guideline production, validation and dissemination were in the hands of a multiplicity of mostly professional agencies, and when no statutory authority was charged with their authentication and approval. How does the appearance of the National Institute for Clinical Excellence (NICE) alter this picture?

NICE and guidelines

NICE has been set up to give guidance to the NHS as a whole, to the Government and ultimately to patients in three broad areas, one of which is appraisal of clinical guidelines (NHS Executive 1999). According to the DoH Memorandum setting out ground rules under which NICE is to operate (DoH 1999b), the Institute will follow a transparent and well-structured process for its appraisals, giving appropriate interested parties the opportunity to submit evidence and to comment on draft conclusions. Appeal to an independent panel will be possible in cases where NICE is alleged to have failed to act fairly, to have exceeded its powers, or to have acted perversely in the light of the evidence submitted.

The Memorandum also conceptualises the Department's view of the legal status of NICE guidance in the following terms:

> 'All guidance must be fully reasoned and written in terms which makes clear that it is guidance. Guidance for clinicians does not override their professional responsibility to make the appropriate decision in the circumstances of the individual patient, in consultation with the patient or guardian/carer and in the light of any locally agreed policies. Similarly, guidance to NHS trusts and commissioners must make clear that it does not take away their discretion under administrative law to take account of individual circumstances' (ibid., p.4).

But despite these caveats, NICE has been charged with ensuring that the implications of its recommendations are carried through to:

- related clinical guidelines;
- PRODIGY guidelines;
- the National Electronic Library for Health;
- protocols used by NHS Direct and NHS Walk-in Centres;
- any material for patients produced by NHS Direct Online.

The DoH clearly views NICE as being structurally and strategically positioned at the hub of a series of influential initiatives and mechanisms designed to facilitate implementation of guidance. How realistic, therefore, is the Department's simultaneously held view that NICE-approved guidance should not be thought to undercut or override clinicians' professional responsibility to make appropriate decisions in the circumstances of the individual patient?

In *R* v *Secretary of State for Health* ex parte *Pfizer Ltd* (1999) the lawfulness of Health Service Circular 1998/158, dated 16 September 1998, was challenged in the High Court, on the grounds that by effectively excluding Viagra (sildenafil) from being prescribed in the NHS by GPs, the Government had breached certain articles of domestic and European legislation. The circular in question contained the heading '*Material which is for guidance only and aims to share good practice*' and stated that: 'The Standing Medical Advisory Committee has advised that doctors should not prescribe sildenafil. Health authorities are also advised not to support the provision of sildenafil at NHS expense to patients requiring treatment for erectile dysfunction, other than in exceptional circumstances' (NHS Executive 1999, p.2).

Counsel for Pfizer, Mr Pannick QC, attacked the lawfulness of the circular on the grounds that, although couched in the terms of advice, its *purpose* and *effect* were to ban, or at the very least, severely to restrict the prescribing of Viagra, to such an extent as to prevent GPs from carrying out their statutory obligations under their Terms of Service in Schedule 2 of the NHS (General Medical Services) Regulations (1992).

In the judge's view: 'The problem with the circular is that the advice was given in a manner which meant that GPs would inevitably regard it as overriding their professional judgement ... To state in bald terms that Viagra should not be prescribed save in (undefined) exceptional circumstances is tantamount to telling the recipients of the advice to follow it' (*R* v *Secretary of State for Health* ex parte *Pfizer Ltd* 1999, p.20).

This judgment is currently being appealed, but what the judge is saying here is that the circular in question was advice in presentation only; in substance and effect it was a directive.

These developments strain credibility in the model hitherto construed to characterise physician-guideline relationships, which posits doctors as free agents, capable of appropriately taking advantage of authoritative guidance without entering into a relationship of professional *reliance* upon guideline guidance. But as the legal analysis of Health Service Circular 1998/158 has shown, executive implementation of authoritative guidance carries with it a danger that guidance can be all too easily packaged as (and therefore mistaken for) instructions. If this happens, it will undermine the ability of clinicians to act as 'master editors' of advisory information, able to modify, and 'pick and mix' guideline advice, blending this advice with that from local treatment policies in an exercise of professional discretion.

Whether or not the kite mark, 'approved by NICE', is likely fundamentally to alter the *title to be believed* of a guideline – its validity, reliability and clinical applicability – such an imprimatur will inevitably carry with it a new kind of warranty, an executive authority not hitherto possessed by previous guidance statements. This warranty stems not only from the methods of appraisal and consultation which NICE adopts – the personnel involved in guideline authentication, their working practices, and how robust adopted guidelines prove to be – but from its structural position within the NHS, which places it in a special relationship with the NHS Executive. In circumstances such as these, where authentication of a guideline entails an executive implementation strategy, NICE guidelines may well constitute guidance which professionals have no choice but to take account of; and failure to do so is likely to be viewed (at the very least) as a serious breach of moral duty.

A culture of compliance

It remains to be seen whether NICE-approved guidelines will attain a new and distinctive legal title to be believed. If they do, deviation from such guidelines may not, in future, merely be viewed as deviation from one approved practice, and fall to be judged according to criteria adopted in the influential Scottish case of *Hunter* v *Hanley* (1955), in which Lord Clyde enunciated criteria for deciding at what point deviation from normal medical practice should be considered negligent. Instead, an action involving failure to consider and/or to adhere to a NICE guideline (where it is alleged a patient has suffered harm as a result) may no longer depend upon a plaintiff having to prove that the care provided fell below the minimum standard required, by calling expert witnesses to testify that no ordinary practitioner acting with ordinary skill would have ignored such a guideline. In cases where a NICE guideline has been ignored, the burden of proof might shift, so that it would be for the defendant doctor to show to the court's satisfaction that the care provided met the required common law standard, notwithstanding failure to apply a NICE guideline (Harpwood 1994).

A pervasive implementation strategy such as the one envisaged for NICE guidelines additionally calls into question the current legal position, whereby guideline authors enjoy a degree of immunity from liability for the production and dissemination of guidelines which may later transpire to be faulty. Generally, there can be no duty of care between the authors of a document or book, and its many readers, unless the authors could foresee that their written advice would be *relied* upon directly, *without independent enquiry*. Prior to the arrival of NICE, clinical guidelines were most unlikely to be deemed to possess sufficient authority for such a claim to be sustained (Hurwitz 1998).

However, Sir Michael Rawlins, chairman of NICE, has now indicated that deviations from NICE-approved guidelines are likely to require greater mental and documentary efforts by clinicians than adherence, and could set in train numerous requests for justification. Vivienne Nathanson, Head of the Science, Ethics and Policy Unit of the British Medical Association, has advised that in circumstances where it is thought NICE guidelines are not applicable for particular patients, doctors are advised 'to record their treatment decisions in the patient's notes to show that they have considered the guidelines' (Jones 1999, p.400).

Clinical guidelines and product liability

Clinical guidelines developed according to more or less formalised and validated techniques, incorporated into software and made available on-line in the consultation, now amount to highly fabricated types of expert advice, distributed in legally tangible forms (Reed 1996). Under common law, a medical appliance or drug requires to be competently designed and manufactured, accompanied by warnings and directions which allow foreseeable users to use it safely (Kennedy & Grubb 1994). Defects in construction or design are actionable. Under the Consumer Protection Act 1987 anyone who suffers injury as a result of a defective product can seek to impose liability upon its producers, manufacturers and those who have brand-named the product (Brazier & Murphy 1999).

If product liability laws could be brought to bear upon clinical guidelines, greater attention would be paid to the guideline/end-user interface than hitherto; and attention would turn to the impact guideline technology has on clinical mentality and discretion within current health care settings. European Directive 93/42/EEC imposes a duty upon manufacturers to prove that devices are fit for the functions for which they are intended, and applies specifically to medical devices. The Directive covers instruments, apparatus, material or other articles intended to be used on human beings for the diagnosis, prevention, monitoring or alleviation of disease, which do not achieve their principal intended actions by using pharmacological, immunological or metabolic means (and includes software necessary) (Harpwood 1998). If clinical guidelines are judged to be within its purview, the Directive will further intensify the need to understand guideline and user interaction.

Summary

Hitherto, courts in the UK have taken note of guidelines (*In re A and others* 1991), have sometimes called for their development and adoption (*Re F* 1989), *over-ruled* prestigious guidelines (*Re W* 1992), and ruled on whether adherence to, or deviation from, specific guidelines was reasonable in particular circumstances (*Loveday* v *Renton and Wellcome Foundation Ltd* 1990; *Re W* 1992; *Early* v *Newham Health Authority* 1994).

UK legal cases have not tended to credit guidelines with a special 'self-evident' status as regards their legal value, and have not adopted standards of care advocated by guidelines, without first evaluating their authority, applicability and the extent to which they represent customary practice. The creation of NICE, with its dual role of supplying special warranty to clinical guidelines and activating an extensive programme of implementation, is likely to result in NICE-approved guidelines being credited with a new and distinctive title to be believed from a legal point of view.

The moral value and conceptual usefulness of treating guidelines and statements of clinical guidance as *manufactured products* which carry, more or less explicitly (or by implication), a quality warranty has been alluded to. If product liability were to attach to the development and warranty of clinical guidelines, the current legal position which offers a degree of immunity from liability to guideline authors might well change. In addition to exposing authors and sponsors of clinical guidelines to increased liability, such a change would promote more intensive consideration of the crucial interface that subsists between guideline and user, which remains currently untheorised and poorly understood.

References

Bolam v *Friern Hospital Management Committee* (1957). *All England Reports* 2, 118–28.

Brazier M & Murphy J (eds) (1999). *Street on torts.* 10th edn. Butterworths, London, pp.337–56.

Department of Health (1999a). *Drug misuse and dependence – guidelines on clinical management.* Department of Health, London.

Department of Health (1999b). *Memorandum of understanding on appraisal of health interventions.* Department of Health, London, 13 Aug.

Early v *Newham Health Authority* (1994). 5 *Med LR* 215–17.

Field M & Lohr K (ed.) (1990). *Clinical practice guidelines: directions for a new programme.* National Academy Press, Washington, DC, USA. 8, 14.

General Medical Council (1998). *Maintaining good medical practice.* GMC, London.

Harpwood V (1994). NHS reform, audit, protocols and standards of care. *Medical Law International* **1**, 241–59.

Harpwood V (1998). *Medical negligence and clinical risk: trends and developments.* Monitor Press, Sudbury, p.40.

Hunter v *Hanley* SC 200 (Court of Session) (1955). Quoted in: Kennedy I & Grubb A (1989). *Medical law. Text and materials.* Butterworths, London, p.420.

Hurwitz B (1998). *Clinical guidelines and the law: negligence, discretion and judgment.* Radcliffe, Abingdon.

In re A and others (minors) (child abuse: guidelines) (1991). 1 *Weekly Law Reports* 1026–32.

Jones J (1999). Influenza drug to undergo 'fast track' assessment by NICE. *BMJ* **319**, 400.

Kennedy I & Grubb A (1994). *Medical law: text with materials.* Butterworths, London, pp.694–708

Lord Scarman (1987). Law and medical practice. In *Medicine in contemporary society* (ed. P Byrne), p.132. King Edward's Hospital Fund for London, London.

Loveday v *Renton and Wellcome Foundation Ltd* (QBD) (1990). 1 *Med LR* 117–204.

Montgomery J (1997). *Health care law.* Oxford University Press, Oxford.

NHS Executive (1996). *Clinical guidelines.* NHS Executive, Leeds.

NHS Executive (1999). Health Service Circular 1999/176. NHS Executive, Leeds.

NHS (General Medical Services) Regulations SI (1992) (as amended); 635: 83–4,138.

Norton-Taylor R (1995). Half the picture. In *Truth is a difficult concept.* A Guardian Book, Fourth Estate Ltd, London.

R v *Secretary of State for Health* ex parte *Pfizer Ltd* (1999). Case No CO/4934/98 High Court of Justice, Queen's Bench Division, May 1999 at 20–25.

Re F (mental patient: sterilisation) (1989). 2 *All England Reports* 545.

Re W (a minor) (1992). 3 *Weekly Law Reports* 758–82.

Reed C (ed.) (1996). *Computer law* 3rd edn. Blackstone Press, London, pp.81–103.

Scott R (1996). *Report of the Inquiry into the Export of Defence Equipment and Dual-Use Goods to Iraq and Related Prosecutions.* HMSO, London.

Stern K (1995). Clinical guidelines and negligence liability. In *Clinical effectiveness. From guidelines to cost effective practice* (ed. M Deighan & S Hitch), pp.127–35. Earlybrave Publications Ltd, Brentwood.

Sudlow M & Thomson RG (1997). Clinical guidelines: quantity without quality. *Qual Health Care* **6**, 60–1.

Thomson RG, McElroy H & Sudlow M (1998). Guidelines on anticoagulant treatment in atrial fibrillation in Great Britain: variation in content and implications for treatment. *BMJ* **316**, 509–13.

Chapter 12

The effect of NICE and CHI on scientific and therapeutic innovation

David G Grahame-Smith

Introduction

It would be a serious matter if measures at policy level designed to improve the quality, availability and cost-effectiveness of patient care inhibited scientific and therapeutic innovation. Should scientific and investigative enthusiasm be stifled by controls which resulted in current practice being embalmed in amber, medical progress would cease.

No one can predict with certainty what impact the National Institute for Clinical Excellence (NICE) and the Commission for Health Improvement (CHI) will have on scientific and therapeutic innovation. My task is to inquire into this potential problem and bring to light those features of the panoply of controls that might have either positive or negative effects upon innovative activity. Anxiety about this in the minds of people involved in innovative activity in the medical sciences should not be dismissed as paranoia.

The effects of controlling the conduct of medicine are difficult to prophesy. Actions intended to do good may do harm: that is common experience. I grant that the Government's actions in producing this control structure spring from the best of motives – to improve the quality of health care delivered to the individual patient and to ensure best use of resources. But along the way has there been no hint that doctors are incompetent and profligate in their use of scarce medical resources and that pharmaceutical companies exist only to provide profits for their shareholders? Let us hope that the motives behind this control structure are free of such prejudices, which I believe are misconceived.

The majority of doctors are neither incompetent nor foolhardy in their use of resources. Although the pharmaceutical industry is capitalist, currently so is our society. The pharmaceutical industry needs vast capital to develop new drugs. The time taken from conception to marketing of an innovative new drug is about 12 years – leaving in Europe eight years of patent life – at a cost of about £150 million. It is a very risky business because a potential new drug can fail at any point along the development process. Those R&D costs for the successes and failures have to be recouped with, naturally, add-on profit within the patent time of a successful drug, by selling the drug at an appropriate cost (regulated by and negotiated with the Government in the UK through the Prescription Price Regulation Scheme for the NHS). The R&D costs of the next drug have to be funded from the profits of the last.

NICE, CHI, National Service Frameworks and clinical governance[1]

When I first heard of the strategic intent to create NICE I cheered, and when I heard that Sir Michael Rawlins was to be its chairman, I cheered again. I thought that NICE was going to do what I, as chairman of our local Drugs and Therapeutics Committee, together with numerous colleagues on that committee, had been trying to do for the last 25 years: to encourage rational prescribing and contain drug costs locally in and around the Oxford hospitals. Untold hours of work have gone into that process all around the country and for years I have wanted to see the process centralised in a body with respected authority. In my *laissez-faire*, namby-pamby, liberal way, I had assumed that NICE would produce guidelines on treatment and that we in the field would be allowed to adapt those to local use and otherwise get on as before, each Drugs & Therapeutics Committee saving a great deal of time from not having to do its own appraisal. The sting comes not from NICE but from national service frameworks (NSFs), CHI and clinical governance, which I think (from what I have read, some of it lacking clarity) are going to make sure 'we' toe the line through formal inspection and audit procedures.

I was also a little surprised to see that NICE will examine the efficacy (and presumably safety) and cost-effectiveness of treatments, using acceptable comparators from current best practice *at a very early stage* of a drug's marketed life, i.e. possibly from launch. Indeed, the University of Birmingham will have a 'horizon-scanning group' to tell NICE what is coming up on the drug development front so that it can prepare itself for 'battle'. I do sympathise. Getting your mind round an innovative new drug therapy, deciding criteria for efficacy, thinking about best usage, seeking most appropriate target groups of patients, deciding on best comparators, guessing about the likely cost burden to the NHS and the level of cost-effectiveness, so that advice can be given in the immediate post-launch phase, are going to be very difficult tasks indeed. If the whole process – NICE, CHI, NSFs, clinical governance – is applied at the launch phase with too heavy a dirigiste hand, there will be tears on four sides, i.e. medical profession, pharmaceutical industry, Government and patients. I would urge during these early stages of establishing a *modus operandi* for NICE and, for its control arms, a light touch.

My hesitation about this early interventionist role of NICE comes from long experience in clinical pharmacology and drug therapy, 12 years on the Committee on Safety of Medicines, an appreciation of the unfolding of the complexities of drug therapy after launch, and experience of being wrong too many times on matters which seemed crystal-clear from the scientific point of view *at the time*. With new drugs, one sometimes has to invent new science! Witness the rocky initial introduction of ACE inhibitors for the treatment of heart failure, the difficulties with xamoterol in heart failure, the long haul to get lithium prophylaxis in manic depressive disease correct, and the development of the astounding prophylactic role of HMG co-A reductase inhibitors in coronary artery disease. In each case new medical science had

---

1. The information upon which my understanding of NICE is based is found in NHS Executive (1999), Department of Health (1999) and on the NICE website (www.nice.org.uk).

to unfold over a period of a few years for us to get a true perspective on these treatments. If at launch these treatments had been preserved in amber, subsequent medical progress would have been deterred.

You may think that NICE will know things of which the medical and pharmaceutical scientific community will be ignorant, but of course it will not. NICE will be trapped by the same confines of medical and scientific knowledge as the rest of us but, because of its bureaucratic foundation and its 'responsibilities for today', it will be less likely to think the unthinkable and profess innovative thought.

NICE will have to tread carefully on treatments at launch. Medicines will already have a product licence from the licensing authority (i.e. the ministers of health) certifying efficacy, safety and the pharmaceutical quality of the product. The granting of product licence is the end of a long process (see Figure 12.1). The point at which NICE will come in is still not clear to me.

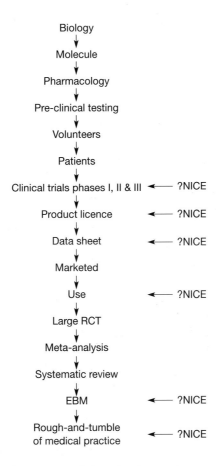

Figure 12.1 Stages in the process of drug development

Horizon-scanning is an art as well as a science. It is possible sometimes to detect at a very early stage (e.g. a receptor interest) that a company is in the business of a new innovative pharmacological area. This requires quite sophisticated pharmacological understanding. I guess and hope that NICE will not involve itself here. It is much more likely to begin being interested during the clinical trials stage. But all those data are going to be 'commercial in confidence' until product licence is granted. If the company wants to let NICE have the data before the licence is granted, all well and good. I guess it might want to, in order to have quick and unhindered access to the UK NHS market through the NICE decision.

I am going into these details because they will determine the speed of appraisal of a new drug by NICE. The appraisal process and its timescale were published by NICE on 6 August 1999. To be absolutely fair to the Department of Health and NICE, there are repeated declarations in NICE's public documentation stating that it is not the Government's intention that the appraisal process should add extra burden on innovators or delay the point at which innovations can be introduced into clinical practice (presumably meaning 'used in the NHS'). But there is a proviso in the documentation: 'provided of course that all parties are able to meet the proposed time scales'. In Appendix C of the NICE guidance document there is a diagrammatic representation of the appraisal process (summarised in Figure 10.2). This is clear for technologies already in use, where the main object is to collect together and summate a considerable amount of information, much of it probably already digested by specialist groups. But for new innovative technologies, the way the process will operate is still not clear to me.

Will NICE, through intelligence obtained by the horizon-scanning group, be approaching pharmaceutical companies for information about their products well before launch date? My reading suggests it will.

Can we be assured that the MCA/CSM axis will truly act independently of NICE? Will there be no collusion and therefore no contrived hold-ups? The reason I raise these concerns is that the licensing system operates under the law, the Medicines Act. There are very strict rules governing the licensing procedure. Licensing of a drug depends strictly upon pharmaceutical quality, efficacy and safety. Comparators are not taken into account (except in respect of relative safety); cost-effectiveness is not an issue; and relative efficacy in special groups of patients as a cost issue is not considered: all such matters are now to be considered by NICE. So, in practice, there are now two big hurdles, rather than one, for new drugs to jump.

The guidance which has been issued indicates that NICE will ask for evidence on clinical effectiveness, cost-effectiveness and the wider NHS implications for new technologies, including drugs, three months before that evidence is to be submitted.

From submission, the appraisal will take a maximum of eight months to run its course, including appeals etc. That is, of course, if all goes smoothly, which it won't. There are going to be serious differences of opinion based upon uncertainties in the

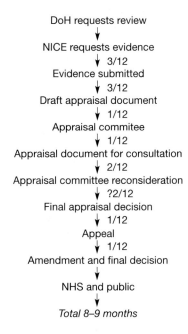

DoH requests review
↓
NICE requests evidence
↓ 3/12
Evidence submitted
↓ 3/12
Draft appraisal document
↓ 1/12
Appraisal commitee
↓ 1/12
Appraisal document for consultation
↓ 2/12
Appraisal committee reconsideration
↓ ?2/12
Final appraisal decision
↓ 1/12
Appeal
↓ 1/12
Amendment and final decision
↓
NHS and public
↓
Total 8–9 months

Figure 12.2 NICE appraisal process

system. Cost-effectiveness can be juggled by health economists, quality of care depends on points of view. Even which patients benefit will be contentious in the early phase of drug introduction into practice.

So there will be a to-and-fro, and it is surely going to take longer than eight months and more than 20 in-house staff to process 20–30 technologies per year (presumably decisions will not be able to be made out of house).

The documentation suggests that if NICE is dissatisfied with the extent of the data available to enable it to reach a decision, it may ask for, or commission, further research. That will prolong the procedure very considerably and I cannot see how that is going to work in practice regarding the speed of decision.

I have described what I understand to be the processes and I accept the excellent role that NICE will have in tidying up technologies already on the market. For example, at the time of writing, NICE was appraising hip prostheses, hearing aids, coronary artery stents, taxanes, proton pump inhibitors in dyspepsia, interferon beta in multiple sclerosis – all technologies where a summation of knowledge can reasonably be made.

The recent appraisal of Relenza (zanamivir), an antiviral for the treatment of influenza, caused some controversy. I believe the claim submitted to NICE was for the treatment of patients in high-risk groups. NICE decided the data were insufficient to support that claim and prescription of the drug on the NHS has not yet been allowed.

Implications for the pharmaceutical industry

In the pharmaceutical industry time is money. Currently, at launch, the company must have available trained medical representatives and all the marketing paraphernalia, systems of some sort of post-marketing surveillance for extent of use, folklore of effectiveness, adverse reaction collection, a trained intelligence network to pick up the unexpected, and an educational system for prescribers. I do not know how the pharmaceutical industry is going to schedule its post-launch activities if it is going to have to wait an uncertain eight months before it can market the drug to the NHS. Drug development has an impetus: a new drug launch, after a 12-year gestatory period, is for the company and its staff an exciting, stimulating experience. Having been granted a product licence, there is now going to be an eight-month delay to uptake of the drug by the NHS, which, like it or not, will be perceived as imposed by DoH bureaucracy. The delay will also eat into patent life. Delays in appraisal, delays through bureaucracy, attitudes of grudging acceptance of submissions, all will adversely effect the morale of innovators.

The negative influences on scientific and therapeutic innovation

I perceive several potential drawbacks to the NICE system, which might have a negative influence on scientific and medical innovation. They include the following:

- bureaucratic delays in the appraisal process;
- the pedantry of an appraisal system unable to come to terms with uncertainty and having to 'watch its back' politically, which will lead to excessive to-ing and fro-ing between sponsor and NICE;
- a system perceived to be grudging in its appraisal attitude such that it appears to resent the advent of certain new technologies;
- mistakes in appraisal. With the best will in the world, at the early introduction of a new medicine, the scientific and medical uncertainties surrounding it are often incapable of speedy resolution. Further experience in the use of the drug in medical practice is needed to determine its real place in therapy, experience which may be difficult to obtain before launch. This may lead to mistakes in appraisal, which will then lead to disrespect for the system and subsequent conflict. There is, for instance, in the documentation produced by NICE, little or no mention of benefit:risk considerations which is a major problem in respect of many new treatments, and which often cannot be fully resolved until many thousands of patients have received the drug in the rough and tumble of everyday medical practice;
- it appears that NICE may ask for further research to be done to answer its questions or commission research from the NHS R&D department. This will inevitably lead to further and considerable delay. It will also lead to companies trying to second-guess the requirements of NICE, which will take up Company time and resources.

Positive influences on scientific and therapeutic innovation

But not all is gloom. NICE will provide authoritative guidelines and advice to aid the use of new technologies and drugs, which should improve the quality and cost-effectiveness of prescribing, and should obviate geographical inequalities in prescribing. It could be that in some instances it will speed the availability of treatments throughout the NHS, but I am less optimistic about that. In time it will remove ineffective treatments from medical practice. These are features of the system which will be seen as spurs to innovation.

I do earnestly hope that in 5–10 years' time it will have created a reputation such that it will be looked to as the arbiter in all matters therapeutic.

The immediate future

NICE has published a list of technologies and drug treatments it will begin to consider in the autumn of 1999 and early in 2000. All of them seem very reasonable topics for consideration. I am also impressed by the reasons for choosing them, though in respect of Cox-2 inhibitors, the influenzal antivirals, anti-obesity treatments, ribavarin and interferon alpha in hepatitis C, treatments for Alzheimer's disease, the glitazones in diabetes, and the glycoprotein IIb/IIIa receptor inhibitors in coronary artery syndromes, the omission of reference to cost-effectiveness and resource implications is less than straightforward. Cost to the NHS is clearly an important factor for all of these treatments.

Conclusions

The UK's drug market share is only 5 per cent or less of the world's market so the controls being put in place there are not going to have a significant impact on the development of drugs at a global level. However, the UK market and its regulatory climate are highly respected in the world, and it will not do a drug or technology any good if its use is severely restricted in the UK, particularly if the sponsoring company is a UK company. Additionally, it is likely that because of increasing cost-containment pressures on health care budgets worldwide, similar controls to those now in place in the UK will be introduced elsewhere.

The motives for scientific and therapeutic innovation run deeper than profit. If a really effective new product reaches the market, no Canute will be able to stem the tide for its use. The clamour of patients and doctors will drive its introduction into the NHS. So there is no real danger to the really effective innovative drug, the use of which is clear. The enthusiasm, morale and excitement which drives major scientific, medical and therapeutic innovation is not going to be dampened by the controls discussed above.

However, I do have concern for the development of 'me-too' drugs which have only little or no advantage over existing treatment (unless they are considerably cheaper!). I am also concerned for those innovative drugs which do not, on the surface, look much better at launch than existing treatments. I suspect they will come under close scrutiny by NICE. Some might not care about that, but I do. Small advances embodied in the pharmacological properties of what at first looks like a 'me-too' drug can, in time, prove very useful and stimulate further research. For example, the newer calcium blockers, HMG co-A reductase inhibitors, SSRIs and newer neuroleptics all belong to classes of drugs where small differences in pharmacology have eventually turned out to have significant therapeutic benefit.

NICE and CHI will have to be very enlightened to understand the potential of such technologies and drugs. If they are not allowed, their development will be inhibited and some small advances that could lead to a major breakthrough might be prevented.

References

Department of Health (1999). *National Institute of Clinical Excellence. Proposed initial work programme and methods of working.* Health Service Circular 1999/176 and Press Release 6 August 1999 (0485).

NHS Executive (1999). *Faster access to modern treatment. A discussion paper.* NHSE, Leeds.

Index